Weekend Doctor

A Reference Guide to Foot Conditions & Treatments

As documented in 'The Courier' Newspaper

by Dr. Thomas F. Vail, DPM

Step Alive Center of Excellence
1725 Western Avenue, Suite C
Findlay, OH 45840
Phone: (419) 423-1888
Fax: (419) 425-3668

www.vailfoot.com

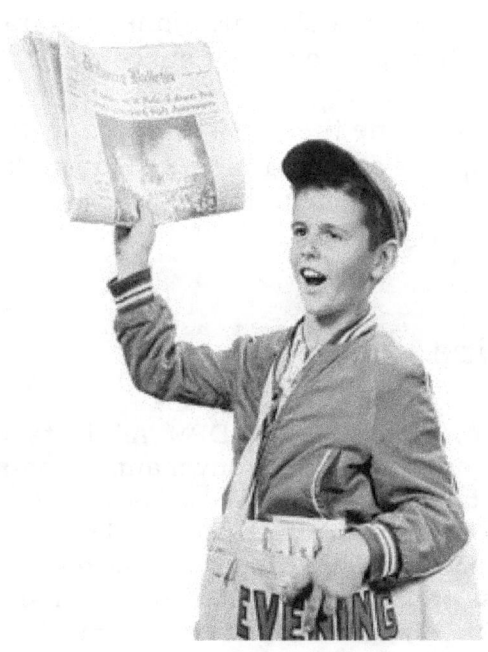

About the Author: Dr. Thomas F. Vail, DPM

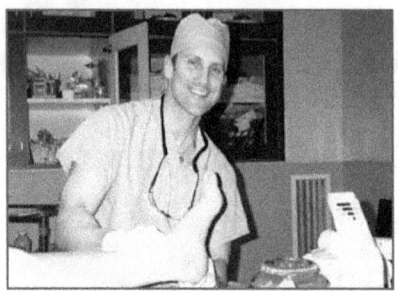

I would like to take this opportunity to introduce myself to you. I am a native of Cleveland, Ohio. As a cum laude graduate of Xavier University in Cincinnati, Ohio, I received my medical degree (DPM) at the Ohio College of Podiatric Medicine in Cleveland, Ohio. My surgical residency was completed in Youngstown, Ohio, with an additional year in South Bend, Indiana, specializing in minimal incision technologies.

I am currently on staff at Blanchard Valley Regional Health Center in Findlay and Bluffton as well as the Findlay Surgery Center. A member of the American Podiatric Medical Association and its Ohio Affiliate, I also am board certified by the American Board of Foot And Ankle Surgery (ABFAS). And I am a Fellow of the American College of Foot and Ankle Surgeons.

My principles have always been to incorporate the latest in care and surgical techniques. The first to introduce Shockwave Therapy for heel pain in Hancock County, I seek out the newest techniques on the horizon for my patients. APC blood platelet injections are another alternative therapy for heel pain that has had great success.

My staff and I would welcome the opportunity to further share with you in person our philosophies and treatments. Our main objective has always been and will continue to be to provide the best quality foot treatment for our patients.

Copyright Notice

Copyright © 2014 by Dr. Thomas F. Vail, DPM. All rights reserved. No part of this book may be used or reproduced in any manner whatsoever without written permission of the author. No expressed or implied guarantees have been made or are made by the authors or publisher. Individual results may vary. Neither author nor publisher accept any liability or responsibility to any person with respect to any loss or damage alleged to have been caused by the information in this book. Always seek professional medical advice.

This book was edited and compiled by Joseph Yorey, BA, MA

Table of Contents

Introduction..6

Chapter 1: Athletic Injuries and Tips for Prevention........7

Lisfranc Injuries in Professional Athletes on the Rise *12-22-12*......................7
New York Yankees Andy Pettitie's Ankle Fracture: Immediate Treatment Essential to Proper Healing *10-6-12*..9
Ice Skating Tips to Prevent Foot Injuries *3-3-12*..............................11
Prevention and Treatment of Ankle Injuries *10-23-10*.........................12
Athlete's and Their Feet *8-1-2009*...14
Runners and Jogger's Foot Pain *7-3-09*.......................................15

Chapter 2: Children's Feet..................................17

Health Issue for Overweight Children *1-22-10*................................17
Back –to- School Children's Feet Tips *8-22-2009*.............................18

Chapter 3: Common Foot Conditions...........................20

Why are My Feet So Puffy? *6-22-13*...20
Is Your Foot Fracture a Sign of Osteoporosis *11-20-10*.......................22
Hammertoes: Can't Touch This! *5-8-10*..23
Got Gout? *1-2-10*..25

Chapter 4: Diabetes and Foot Care...........................27

The Not So Sweet Truth About Peripheral Neuropathy and Diabetes 2 *8-4-12*......27

Chapter 5: Foot Tips.......................................29

Do Rented Bowling shoes Pose a Health Risk? *9-21-13*.........................29
At Odds: Smoking and Foot Surgery *8-3-13*....................................31
Pedicure Tips for the Summer & Beyond *7-13-13*...............................33
Feet Can Hold Clues to Heart Health *4-21-12*.................................34
Foot Tips for Summer Picnics *7-2-11*...36

Travel Tips for Deep Leg Thrombosis *4-16-11*..37
New Year's Resolution Safety Foot Tips at the Gym *1-15-11*..............................38
Five Tips for Healthy Holiday Feet *12-18-10*..40
Seven Myths about Foot Care *9-18-10*..42
Healthy Feet Make the Best Dancing Feet *3-1-10*..44
Beach Barefoot Safety Tips *6-6-09*..46
Eliminate Foot Pain to Lose Weight *4-18-09*..47
Taking a Vacation? Make it Easy on Your Feet! *5-9-09*......................................48

Chapter 6: General Foot Injuries..50

Fractures of the Body can Cause Foot Damage *9-7-13*..50
Achilles Tendon Rupture Treatment *9-10-11*..52
Lawnmowers: Use Caution to Avoid Foot Injuries *5-21-11*................................54
Winter is Fall Season *1-28-10* 55

Chapter 7: Heel Pain..58

Victor Cruz: Not the Only one Affected by Sports Injuries *11-2-13*...................58
APC Injections Can Benefit All Not Just Professional Athletes *5-18-13*.................60
Revolutionary Blood Platelet Injections *12-19-09* 61
Heel Pain & Young Athletes *11-14-09*..63

Chapter 8: Gait Analysis and Correction........................64

The Pain in Your Back Could be Linked to Your Feet *3-23-13*...........................64
Flat Feet: Causes, Surgical Treatments and Beneficial Exercises Q & A *12-1-12*...66
Flatfoot Disorders and Current Treatments *8-20-11*..69
Read Your Footprints and How You Roll *7-3-10*..70

Chapter 9: Men's Foot Health..72

Top 10 Men's Foot Problems and Treatments *2-9-13*...72

Chapter 10: Skin Conditions of the Feet......................75

Diagnosis of Melanoma Saves Lives *11-10-12*...75
Flesh Eating Bacteria and Tips to Save your Feet *7-7-12*...................................77

Chapter 11: Shoes and the Proper Fit.............................79

Flip Flop Injuries in Young Adults *6-16-12*..79
Rock & Roll for Your Feet: Will Toning Shoes Give You That Rockin' Body? *3-5-11*..81
High Heeled Shoe Damage and Simple Tips for Prevention *1-22-11* 83
Back to School Shoe Tips *8-7-10*..86

Chapter 12: Sports and your Feet...............................89

Minnesota Viking's Harrison Smith Sidelined with Turf Toe: Causes & Treatments *12-21-13*..89
Shin Splints…your Feet may be the Culprit! *4-20-13*..91
Bowling and Your Feet *11-12-11*..92
Improve Your Golf Swing by Starting with your Feet *7-23-11*.........................94

Chapter 13: Women's Foot Health..............................96

June Brides see Podiatrists in July for Foot Problems *6-1-13*...........................96
Female Athletes at Risk for Foot & Ankle Injuries During Menstrual Cycle *3-24-12*..98
Enjoy Pregnancy without Foot Pain *3-20-10*...100
Bunions in Women's Feet Worse in Fall Boots *10-3-09*..................................101

Chapter 14: Bonus Section...103
Findlay Footsteps Courier Article, Shoe Recommendations & Exercises

Lace Up and Get Fit: Dr. Vail releases new pictorial book on walking paths in Findlay, Ohio...103
Top Pediatric Shoes...107
Adult Shoe Recommendations..113
Friendly Footwear For Those Who Work Standing Up.....................................117
How to Choose an Athletic Shoe that's Right for You.......................................121
Heel Pain/Plantar Fasciitis Stretching Exercises..124

Introduction

This publication is a compilation of all of Dr. Thomas F. Vail's published Weekend Doctor articles for 'The Courier' newspaper in Findlay, OH. The articles give invaluable insight regarding common foot problems and treatments.

The articles written for this publication by Dr. Vail span the course of 5 years from 2009 thru 2013. The book was designed to give patients a more organized version of all Dr. Vail's articles and the information provided by the popular 'Weekend Doctor' series in the Weekend Edition of the Courier newspaper.

Use this book as a reference for general foot ailments and treatments or just for the times when you simply can't remember where you put that newspaper clipping!

Remember, foot pain is not normal and your podiatrist can get you back to enjoying life's activities again.

Chapter 1

Athletic Injuries and Tips for Prevention

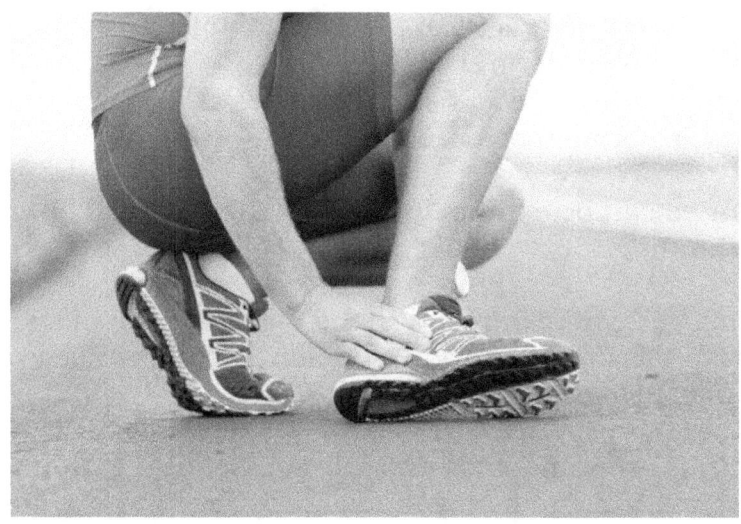

Lisfranc Injuries in Professional Athletes on the Rise

Published: *12-22-12*

At last, football season has come to a close. We have endured the long road with our favorite team. Unfortunately, every season brings the possibility that our favorite player might get injured.

In just one week in October, three NFL players succumbed to foot injuries. New York Jets wide receiver Santonio Holmes, Green Bay Packers running back Cedric Benson, and Carolina Panthers center Ryan Kalil all suffered Lisfranc injuries.

Most of us know about common athletic injuries such as a torn ACL or an ankle sprain. However, with the way this year's football season started, it may be worth your time to learn about Lisfranc injuries.

The Lisfranc joint connects your forefoot to your midfoot. In other words, the Lisfranc joint connects the bones in the front of the foot (toes and metatarsals), to the bones in the middle of the foot (cuneiforms and cuboid). This joint is held in place by several ligaments.

The Lisfranc joint is very important in stabilizing the arch of your foot. A sharp and sudden twisting motion of the foot, like those made when playing football, can cause damage to the Lisfranc ligaments.

Podiatrists usually put Lisfranc injuries into three categories:

- Lisfranc injury: A ligament is stretched (sprained) out of its normal range.
- Lisfranc fracture: A ligament is torn completely and a piece of bone has broken off (fracture).
- Lisfranc fracture dislocation: The bones of the midfoot have shifted from their normal position.

Lisfranc injuries can be extremely painful. The pain will be worse when walking or standing.

Like other injuries, you can rest, ice and elevate the area. However, if you think you have a Lisfranc injury, you definitely want to be evaluated by your podiatrist for a proper diagnosis.

Lisfranc injuries are sometimes difficult to diagnose, so you will need a qualified foot specialist to help you manage your injury. A diagnosis can be made through clinical tests such as the "piano key" test (moving the toes up and down to see where the injury is) or by imaging tests such as X-rays, MRI or CT scan.

The treatment for a Lisfranc injury depends on how severe the injury is. A sprain of the ligament typically requires a cast that is worn for several weeks. A fracture will more than likely need surgical repair.

To completely fix the injury, your podiatrist may need to use wires and screws inside the foot to help your foot stay stable. Whenever you undergo foot surgery, always follow the rehabilitation guidelines set by your podiatrist.

This type of injury can require you to stay off your injured foot for at least six to eight weeks. It may be difficult to stay off your feet for this long, but it is all for the best.

Even with the best care, Lisfranc injuries take a while to completely heal. If you neglect your injury or do not follow rehabilitation guidelines, your chances of having complications are higher.

Complications include chronic pain and early arthritis. Now that you know about Lisfranc injuries, let's hope that our favorite players avoid this foot injury during the upcoming bowl games. And, go Irish!

New York Yankees Andy Pettitte's Ankle Fracture: Immediate Treatment Essential to Proper Healing

Published: *10-6-12*

When a fracture occurs in the foot and ankle, it is important to see a physician immediately for proper diagnosis and treatment. It will help regain complete function of the injury without causing further complications.

Recovery times vary depending on the type of fracture.

A minor bone break may take a few weeks to heal, while a serious break in a bone may require months to as much as a year to heal.

New York Yankees left-hander Andy Pettitte's fractured his left ankle on June 27 and was out for 10 weeks. He started simulated game/live batting practice against hitters on Sept. 5.

The 40-year-old Pettitte was hit on the ankle by a line drive in the fifth inning of a game against the Cleveland Indians. The Yankees said Pettitte healed without needing surgery.

Foot or ankle fractures should always be treated as well as the patient following up with a doctor to make sure that no other problems exist such as displacement of bone or dislocations.

Mistaking an ankle fracture for an ankle sprain also has serious consequences when the foot does not heal correctly. You should always seek the correct diagnosis to ensure proper recovery.

An ankle fracture involves a crack or break in the bones that form the ankle joint. A sprain involves the ligaments that hold the ankle bones together. Both injuries can happen simultaneously when the ankle moves beyond its normal range of motion, but a fracture requires more complex treatment than a sprain.

Sprains are so commonplace people want to believe that is what is going on, but prolonged pain and bruising should trigger awareness that it might not be just a sprain. Having pain but still being able to walk is not a good test to determine if it's a sprain or a fracture because walking is still possible with less-severe injuries.

Signs of a fracture include bruising, blisters, significant swelling or bone protruding through the skin. In addition to bone, ankle fractures can also involve cartilage surrounding the bones.

Patients with unrecognized ankle fractures have a high risk of developing infection, arthritis and foot deformities that may make it impossible to walk normally again.

It is imperative that patients with diabetes, vascular disease, alcoholism and immune deficiency receive prompt care from a foot and ankle surgeon because they are extremely vulnerable to nerve damage, infection and Charcot Foot, a very serious condition that can lead to foot deformity, disability, or even amputation.

Proactive prevention is crucial to avoid ankle injuries, including a good foot assessment and using canes or walkers for stability. I also advise buying from small shoe stores that have certified orthotists and shoe fitters who work with foot and ankle surgeons and assess if shoes and insoles support patients' feet correctly.

Incidents of ankle fractures in children, teenagers and young men are increasing mainly due to elite athletics.

Fractures need to be monitored so bones fuse together correctly and don't affect the foot's growth plate, a strip of new bone in pediatric patients that grows as feet lengthen. If the growth plate is damaged, it could produce bone spurs and arthritis, and pre-maturely halt bone growth.

Improved therapies and surgical approaches continue to offer solutions for complicated cases and produce better results, and are available to a wider range of patients:

- Total ankle replacements, similar to hip and knee replacements, were once reserved for geriatric patients but are now used in younger patients.
- Screws and other fasteners to bind bone and cartilage dissolve inside the body so second surgeries to remove them are not necessary.

- Newly developed synthetic and natural grafting materials are used in ankle repair when optimal healing would not otherwise occur.
- Small devices worn externally are now used to stimulate bone growth using pulsed ultrasound and electromagnetic fields.

So let's learn from Andy Pettitte's ankle fracture and seek immediate care and diagnosis with your podiatrist for any ankle problems to prevent further complications

Ice Skating Tips to Prevent Foot Injuries

Published: *3-3-12*

Ice skating is an excellent way to enjoy the winter weather and get some exercise. But ice skating can quickly lose its appeal if your feet begin to hurt.

Ice skating and ice skates are associated with several common foot ailments including calluses, blisters and ankle problems. Because of the risks ice sports pose with falling, it is important for skaters to purchase the proper shoe for the activity they will be doing.

It is also important to be fit by a trained professional whenever buying a new pair of skates.

Hockey skates are made to move, turn and stop quickly on the ice. The skate has a curved shape and a hollow blade. This helps the skater with speed and agility.

A figure skate has a toe pick, curved blade, long blade and leather boots. These features help the figure skater to execute jumps, turns and deep knee bends.

Figure skaters need to be especially careful when they are told to point their toes. Most skaters will scrunch up their toes, causing the calf muscle to shorten. If the skater points their foot by extending the ankle, it is much easier on the calf muscle and the knee will straighten with more ease.

For those who have never been ice skating, a figure skate is a good option. The blade allows you to distribute your weight evenly.

Be sure to wear protective socks to avoid blisters. Skaters should also make sure the skates fit properly before getting on the ice. Try these tips when buying your next pair of skates:

1. Most people have different size left and right feet. Have your feet measured and buy skates to fit your bigger foot.
2. When you measure the length of your feet, make sure you are using the heel-to-ball measurement. This measurement is the most accurate measurement to determine proper length.
3. The proper width measurement of your feet is made by sliding the brannock device to touch the edge of the foot. If a foot has a high instep, it may be necessary to fit an extra width wider. This is where the expertise of your shoe fitting specialist comes into play.
4. Bring the type of socks you will be wearing with your skates. Socks will affect the fit of the boot, especially thick winter socks.
5. Every brand of skates fits differently. Make sure you try on several different brands before deciding on which fits best.
6. Lace the boots firmly with most of the pressure at the top four eyelets. A secure fit is very important.

Boots that are too soft or too stiff can cause several problems and slow down your axels and slap shots. Boots that are too stiff can cause Achilles injury or tendonitis. Boots that are too loose can cause Haglund's deformity, a boney enlargement on the back of the heel.

Remember, foot pain is not normal when you skate. Keep a few second-skin pads and gel pads on hand at your next skating event so you can eliminate the blisters and calluses afterward.

If you are experiencing any of these problems or any problems with your feet and ankles, don't hesitate to see your podiatrist.

Prevention and Treatment of Ankle Injuries

Published: *10-23-10*

Every fall, I notice an increase in ankle injuries among young athletes. Football, soccer and basketball are the sports most likely to lead to sprains, broken bones and other problems. My top recommendation is for parents to get ankle injuries treated right away.

What seems like a sprain is not always a sprain. In addition to cartilage injuries, your son or daughter might have injured other bones in the foot without knowing it.

Have a qualified doctor examine the injury. The sooner rehabilitation starts, the sooner we can prevent long-term problems like instability or arthritis, and the sooner your child can get back into competition. Parents should follow these additional tips: Have old sprains checked by a doctor before the season starts.

A medical check-up can reveal whether your child's previously injured ankle might be vulnerable to sprains, and could possibly benefit from wearing a supportive ankle brace during competition. There are some very good supportive ankle braces available now that fit into most athletic shoes. Your podiatrist will be able to recommend the proper brace for your children's condition.

Buy the right shoe for the sport. Different sports require different shoe gear. Players shouldn't mix baseball cleats with football shoes. Children should start the season with new shoes. Old shoes can wear down like a car tire and become uneven on the bottom, causing the ankle to tilt because the foot can't lie flat.

If you see a repetitive wear pattern on the bottom of your children's shoes, they probably would benefit from custom orthotics.

All children can benefit from custom orthotics. Today, custom molded orthotics come in many shapes, sizes and materials that allow people to stand, walk, and run more efficiently and comfortably. While over-the-counter orthotics are available and may help people with mild symptoms, they normally cannot correct the wide range of symptoms that prescription foot orthoses can since they are not custom made to fit an individual's unique foot structure.

Consult your podiatrist on the newest materials for custom orthotics specifically made for your child's particular sport. Check playing fields for dips, divots and holes. Most sports-related ankle sprains are caused by jumping and running on uneven surfaces.

That's why some surgeons recommend parents walk the field, especially when children compete in non-professional settings like public parks, for spots that could catch a player's foot and throw them to the ground. Alert coaching officials to any irregularities. Lastly, encourage stretching and warm-up exercises. Calf stretches and light jogging before a competition helps warm up ligaments and blood vessels, reducing the risk for ankle injuries.

Athletes and their Feet

Published: *8-1-09*

There are several common foot ailments that sports enthusiasts, and others, should watch for.

With more than 250,000 sweat glands in the foot, it's no surprise that foot odor can affect anyone.

Daily hygiene, in addition to the regular changing of socks and shoes, are the best ways to control foot sweat and odor.

Runners should avoid wearing cotton socks and running without socks. Foot powders, aerosols, antiperspirants and vinegar soaks can be helpful in preventing and treating foot odor.

Blisters, corns and calluses can cause problems, but are usually easy to treat.

Never pop blisters unless they are larger than a quarter, painful or swollen.

Use a sterile instrument to lance the corner, leaving the top as a natural, biological dressing. Wash, apply antibiotic ointment and cover with a bandage.

Corns and calluses are caused by repeated friction and should be treated by aseptically trimming the dead skin and eliminating the underlying cause.

Athlete's foot is a fungal skin disorder that causes dry, cracking skin between the toes, itching, inflammation and blisters.

Athlete's foot can be prevented and controlled by:

- washing the feet regularly
- carefully drying between the toes
- switching running shoes every other day to allow them to dry
- wearing socks made with synthetic material instead of cotton

- applying over-the-counter ointments

Ingrown toenails can cause inflammation and possible infection. They are usually treated by cutting the corner of the nail with sterile clippers.

Black toenails happen when trauma causes a blood blister to form under the nail. In this case, it's best to let the nail fall off by itself.

Fungal toenails are yellow, brown or black, and are sometimes irregularly shaped and thick. They are best treated with oral anti-fungal medications that a physician can prescribe.

If you have questions about your feet, whether you're an athlete or not, talk to your podiatrist.

Runners and Jogger's Foot Pain

Published: 7-3-09

Both long-distance runners and casual joggers can improve their performance by keeping their feet in top condition and taking steps to control foot problems common in runners.

The human foot is a biological masterpiece that can endure the stress of daily activity. For runners, the feet are more vulnerable to injury than any other part of the body. Runners should watch for signs of foot problems that can slow them down if not treated promptly.

The most common complaint from runners is heel pain. This condition, also called plantar fasciitis, is frequently caused by inflammation of the ligament that holds up the arch.

Heel pain can result from faulty mechanics and overpronation, when pressure is unequally applied to the inside of the foot. It can also be caused by wearing running shoes that are worn out or too soft.

At the first sign of heel pain, runners should do stretching exercises, wear sturdier shoes and use arch supports. In some cases, icing and anti-inflammatory drugs like ibuprofen can help.

If heel pain continues, custom orthotics, injections or physical therapy might be required. Normally, surgery isn't considered unless heel pain persists for more than a year and conservative treatment fails to bring relief.

Neuromas and tendonitis are other common foot problems that affect runners.

A neuroma is a pinched nerve between the toes that can cause pain, numbness and a burning sensation in the ball of the foot. Overly flexible shoes are often the cause; padding, orthotics or injections are usually effective. Sometimes, surgery is recommended if pain between the toes continues for more than six months.

Serious runners can also be sidelined by tendonitis, as can overzealous beginners who try too much too soon.

There are several forms of tendonitis that affect the Achilles and other areas; all are treated with rest, icing, stretching, anti-inflammatory medications, and sometimes orthotics or physical therapy.

A common myth among athletes is that it's not possible to walk or run if a bone in the foot is fractured.

I often hear surprised patients say, "It can't be broken; I can walk on it." That's dead wrong, especially with stress fractures, when pain and swelling might not occur for a few days.

If a fracture or sprain is suspected, I advise runners to remember the acronym "RICE," referring to rest, ice, compression and elevation.

If pain and swelling continues after following RICE for three or four days, see a foot and ankle surgeon for an X-ray and proper diagnosis.

Chapter 2

Children's Feet

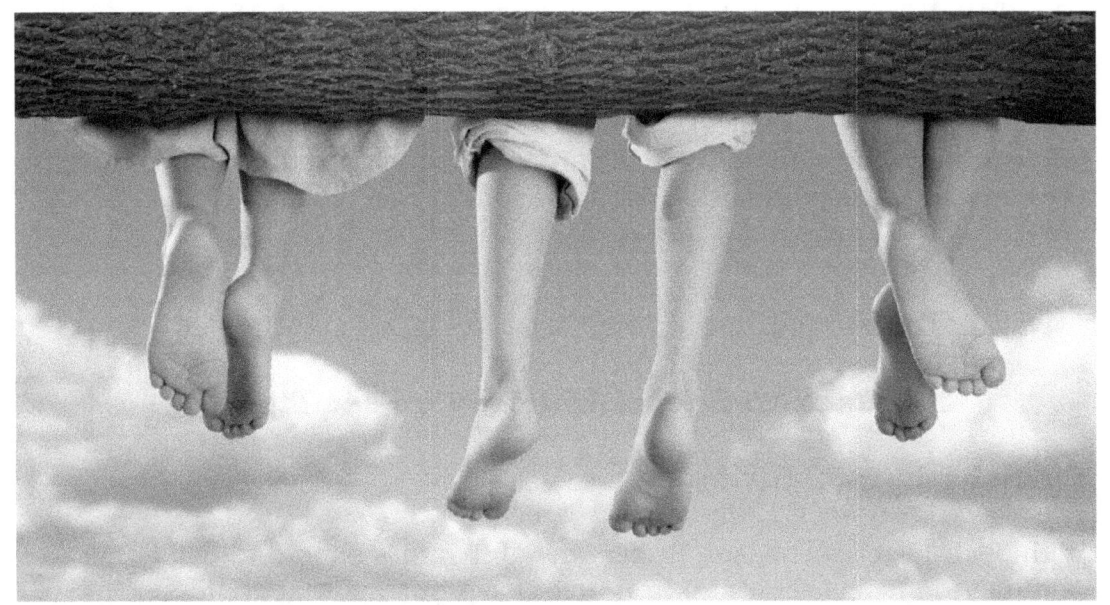

Another Health Issue for Overweight Children

Published: *1-22-10*

Being overweight makes kids' feet hurt... and when their feet hurt they're less active.

It's a "vicious cycle" says Dr. Tom Vail of Findlay's Advanced Foot Care.

"We're seeing more and more obese children with foot and ankle problems," adds Dr. Vail. "You want overweight children to exercise and lose weight, but because of their weight their feet hurt and they can't exercise."

An estimated sixteen percent of U.S. children ages six to nineteen are overweight. Last year, researchers in Britain reported alarming new evidence that childhood obesity actually changes the foot structure and results in instability when walking. Being overweight flattens the foot, straining the plantar fascia, causing heel pain. Those extra child hood pounds can also exacerbate congenital foot conditions like bunions and hammertoes.

Dr. Vail says that he can help reduce foot pain in overweight children with orthotics, physical therapy and other conservative measures; however, he emphasizes that parents need to take responsibility for overseeing their child's lifestyle and diet.

"We can treat the symptoms, but parents need to help their child address the cause of their pain and the real reason for inactivity."

Back-to-School Children's Feet Tips

Published: *8-22-09*

With back to school season underway, all parents should take a few minutes to inspect their children's feet for problems that could sideline their son or daughter from sports or other fall activities.

Parents can spot several potential foot problems by observing how their kids walk.

Parents can ask these questions:

- Does my pre-schooler walk on his or her toes?
- Does my child walk irregularly?
- Is one of my child's legs longer than the other?
- Do my child's feet turn in or out excessively?
- Does my child often trip or stumble?
- Does the bottom of my child's shoes show uneven wear patterns?
- Does my child complain of tired legs, night pains or cramping?

These simple questions can uncover common problems like ingrown toenails or more serious problems.

Some younger children toe-walk because of tightness in their Achilles tendon. This can happen when toddlers spend too much time in walkers. A foot and ankle surgeon can recommend stretching exercises that can be fun for small children and help prevent lower back pain as they get older.

If one of your child's legs is longer than the other, heel lifts may be required to restore proper balance. Early intervention could prevent scoliosis (a curvature of the spine) later in life.

In addition, look at your child's shoes. For example, if a shoe is worn on the big toe side, it could be a sign of poor arch support or flat feet.

Leg and foot pain can indicate flat feet or other disorders that are easier to treat the earlier they are diagnosed. Remember: children with flat feet are at risk for arthritis later in life if the problem is left untreated.

Don't be fooled; growing pains are a myth! If your kids complain about tired legs, heel pain or cramping in their legs or feet at night, consider that a warning sign and see a doctor.

In the fall, I also see many college-age students complaining about pain from walking so much every day. Heel pain and shin splints can plague freshman not used to walking long distances across campus to attend classes.

For most students, daily stretching and proper walking shoes can easily solve this problem. If there are foot deformities like hammertoes, surgery may be advised to make walking more comfortable.

Chapter 3

Common Foot Conditions

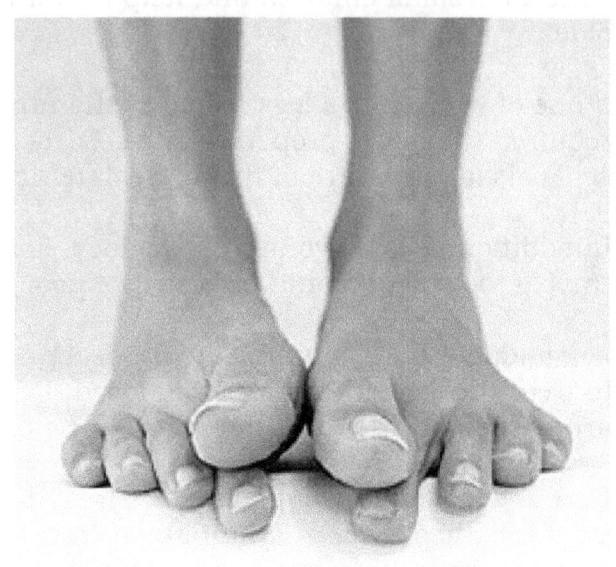

Why Are My Feet So Puffy?

Published: *6-22-13*

Kim Kardashian was recently photographed wearing high heeled sandals. This doesn't seem out of the ordinary except for the fact the Kim is very pregnant with very swollen feet. There was much online talk about Kim's puffy feet and the majority of the comments were not nice. Kim leads a public personal life that most of us can't and don't want to relate to. However, swollen feet and ankles is a common issue for many people.

Excess fluid in the limbs can be very uncomfortable and make wearing properly fitting shoes difficult. Pregnancy is only one cause of swollen limbs. With summer fast approaching, most of us are trading in the long pants for shorts and wearing more revealing shoe gear. Before the weather gets too warm, now is a good time to find out the cause of your swollen feet.

1. **Heart, liver, or kidney disease** – Heart disease is the leading cause of death in the US. Right-sided heart failure is when the right side of your heart isn't pumping blood properly to the lungs and the left side of the heart. Blood builds up in the lower limbs leading to swollen feet and ankles. Fluid also builds up in the legs if the kidneys are diseased and cannot filter fluid properly. The

liver makes a protein called albumin that keeps blood from leaking out of vessels. If the liver is damaged, albumin decreases and fluid begins to accumulate in the ankles and feet.

2. **Venous Insufficiency** – The veins in our legs are one-way valves that bring blood back to the heart. When veins are damaged or weakened, the blood cannot move back toward the heart and stands still. This retained fluid leads to swollen legs, ankles and feet. If nothing is done to push the fluid upward, skin ulcers and infection can occur.

3. **Blood clot** – Blood clots in the legs are very serious. A blood clot in the deep veins of the legs is called a deep vein thrombosis. This type of blood clot can stop blood flow back to the heart and cause swelling in the legs, ankle, and feet. Death can occur if this blood clot breaks off and travels to the heart and lungs. Signs of a deep vein thrombosis are painful swelling in one leg, a low fever, and possibly a change in color of the affected leg. Treatment for deep vein thrombosis involves the use of blood thinners to break up the clot.

4. **Medications** – Finally, many drugs that people take daily can cause swelling in the feet and ankles. The drugs include oral contraceptives, hormone replacement therapy, calcium-channel blockers, steroids, anti-depressants, non-steroidal anti-inflammatory medications and diabetic medication.

There are several more causes for swollen feet and ankles including, injury, infection, thyroid disease, too much salt intake, too much alcohol use, and aging. It is very important to get a correct diagnosis for proper treatment. Some forms of treatment are elevating the legs, dietary changes, stopping medication, protein replacement and wearing compression stockings to bring fluid back towards the heart. Once you know the cause, your podiatrist will help you determine which treatment is best for you.

Kim's swollen feet in high heels may look humorous, but it is not a laughing matter. Swollen feet can be a sign of a more serious problem. Check your feet daily and be sure to schedule an appointment with your podiatrist.

Is Your Foot Fracture a Sign of Osteoporosis?

Published: *11-20-10*

Unexplained foot fractures may be the first sign of osteoporosis, a bone-thinning disease that affects over 28 million Americans and accounts for 1.5 million bone fractures a year.

Osteoporosis is frequently referred to as the "silent crippler" since it often progresses without any symptoms or isn't diagnosed until a person experiences pain from a bone fracture.

The porous nature of bones in people with osteoporosis makes them more susceptible to bone fractures, especially in the feet.

Because the bones are in a weakened state, normal, weight-bearing actions like walking can cause the bones in the feet to break.

In fact, many patients visit their foot and ankle surgeon suffering from foot pain only to find out they actually have a stress fracture without having experienced an injury.

While osteoporosis is most commonly seen in women over age 50, younger people and men are also affected.

Early symptoms can include increased pain with walking accompanied by redness and swelling on the top of the foot.

Often times, patients don't seek treatment for their symptoms for weeks or even months, thinking the pain will pass.

The best advice is to don't ignore foot pain of any type.

Early intervention can make all the difference in your treatment and recovery.

Foot and ankle surgeons are able to diagnose osteoporosis through bone densitometry tests, which measure calcium and mineral levels in the bones through low-dose radiation X-ray, or possibly through a routine X-ray.

This is why prevention and early intervention is the key. Women should make sure bone densitometry tests are part of their wellness examinations when indicated by their physicians.

If you are diagnosed with osteoporosis, it's important to protect your feet from stress fractures.

Wear shoes that provide support and cushioning, such as athletic running shoes, to provide extra shock absorption and protection.

Custom orthotics may also be recommended to protect the foot from pressure and provide shock absorption, particularly during exercise.

Remember that "custom orthotics" are not the same as the "custom fitted" pairs you can buy at your mass retailers today.

Custom orthotics are handmade, individualized orthotics made to a doctor's specifications from a three-dimensional scan or mold of your feet.

Don't be fooled by the "custom fitted" orthotics that are selected after you step on a pressure pad and it places your order. They are packaged and sent to you from a distribution center.

If you are suffering from foot pain or suspect you may have osteoporosis, call your podiatrist for an evaluation.

Hammertoes: Can't Touch This!

Published: 5-8-10

A hammertoe is formed from an abnormal balance of the muscles in the toes.

This causes increased pressures on the tendons and joints of the toe, leading to the contracture or bending of the toe at the first joint of the digit, called the "proximal interphalangeal joint."

This bending causes the toe to appear like an upside-down "V."

Any toe can be involved, but the condition usually affects the second through fifth toes, known as "the lesser digits."

A visit to your podiatrist can be the first step to relief.

First, the podiatrist will determine what type of hammertoes you have.

They could be flexible hammertoes, which are less serious because they can be diagnosed and treated while still developing, or rigid hammertoes, which are more developed and more serious.

Rigid hammertoes can be seen in patients who wait too long to seek professional treatment or in patients with severe arthritis.

The tendons in a rigid hammertoe become tight and the joint misaligned and immobile, making surgery the usual course of treatment.

The treatment options vary with the type and severity of each hammertoe, although identifying the deformity early in its development is important to avoid surgery.

Your podiatric physician will examine and X-ray the affected area and recommend a treatment plan.

Your doctor may recommend:

• Padding and taping, often the first step in a treatment plan. Padding the hammertoe prominence minimizes pain and allows you to continue a normal life. Taping may change the imbalance around the toes and relieve the stress and pain.

• Medication such as anti-inflammatory drugs and cortisone injections to ease acute pain and inflammation caused by the joint deformity.

•Orthotic devices like custom shoe inserts made by your podiatrist, which may be useful in controlling foot function. An orthotic device may reduce symptoms and prevent the worsening of the hammertoe deformity.

If these treatments are not effective, several surgical procedures are also available to the podiatric physician.

For less severe deformities, the surgery will remove the bony prominence and restore normal alignment of the toe joint, which relieves pain.

Severe hammertoes, which are not fully reducible, may require more complex surgical procedures.

Hammertoes are common and don't need to be a pain.

Got Gout?

Published: *1-2-10*

Got gout? If so, watch what you eat and drink. Changes in diet, including overindulging in certain foods and beverages, can cause gout attacks.

Gout, also known as gouty arthritis, is extremely painful. Gout is caused when uric acid accumulates in the tissues or a joint and crystallizes. Gout most commonly occurs in the big toe joint because it is subject to so much pressure from walking. The big toe is also the coolest part of the body and uric acid is sensitive to temperature changes.

Men are more likely to suffer from a gout attack than women. A common symptom of gout is waking up in the middle of the night with a throbbing pain in your big toe, which is swollen.

The pain lasts about three or four hours and then subsides. However, pain in the same toe usually returns within a few months.

So how is gout diagnosed? Your doctor will ask questions about your symptoms and do a physical exam. He or she might take a fluid sample from your joint to look for uric acid crystals, which is the best way to test for gout. Your doctor may also do a blood test to measure the amount of uric acid in your blood. Paying attention to what you eat can help you manage gout. People prone to gout attacks should avoid purine-rich items such as shellfish, organ meats like kidney and liver, red meat, red wine, and beer.

Other protein compounds in foods, such as lentils and beans, may cause gout. Eat moderate amounts of a healthy mix of foods to control your weight and get the nutrients you need. In addition, drink plenty of water and other fluids.

If prevention is not enough, gout can be treated with medications, diet changes, increasing consumption of appropriate fluids, and immobilizing the foot.

If you treat gout right away, relief often begins within 24 hours.

To ease pain during a gout attack, rest the joint that hurts. Apply ice or cooling lotions to your toe to ease pain and swelling during an acute attack.

Taking ibuprofen or another anti-inflammatory medicine can also help you feel better. However, don't take aspirin; it can make gout worse by raising the level of uric acid in your blood. As always, talk to your physician before taking any medications.

To stop a gout attack, your doctor can also give you a shot of corticosteroids, or prescribe a large daily dose of one or more medicines. The doses will get smaller as your symptoms go away.

In some cases, specially-made shoes are prescribed to relieve pain associated with gout.

In severe cases, surgery may be required to remove uric acid crystals and repair the joint.

To prevent future attacks, your doctor may prescribe a medicine to reduce uric acid buildup in your blood.

If your doctor prescribes this medication, take it as directed. Most people continue to take this medicine for the rest of their lives.

Talk to a podiatrist if you have other questions about gout.

Chapter 4

Diabetes and Foot Care

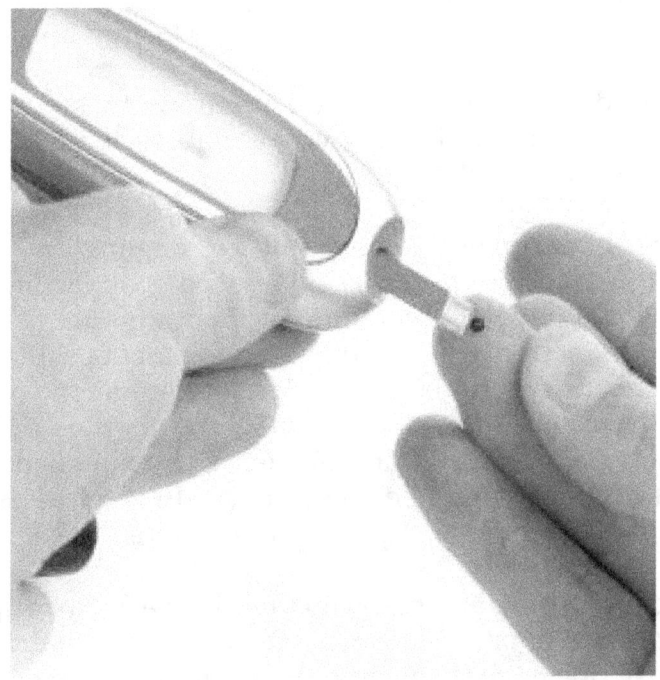

The Not So Sweet Truth About Peripheral Neuropathy

Published: *8-4-12*

Earlier this year, celebrity chef Paula Deen caused controversy when she revealed that she was diagnosed with type 2 diabetes three years ago.

Type 2 diabetes is always in the news, but there is still much that doctors and scientists do not know about the disease. There are several risk factors including obesity, race, age, family history and high blood pressure.

Type 2 diabetes does not have to be an early death sentence. With proper medications and lifestyle changes, diabetics can live an active, enjoyable life.

Once you have been diagnosed with diabetes, you will need to see your primary care physician regularly.

Many people do not know, but the feet can sometimes show the first signs of a diabetic issue.

Peripheral neuropathy is very common in type 2 diabetics. It is when diabetes affects the nerves and a person looses feeling in their feet.

For instance, if a diabetic with peripheral neuropathy stepped on glass, they wouldn't feel the pain. The only way a diabetic would know they were injured, is if they see the wound.

Some early signs of peripheral neuropathy are tingling, burning, itching and sometimes pain in the feet or legs. We need good feeling in our feet. Imagine what would happen if you cut your foot and didn't know it for days or weeks. Unfortunately, this happens to diabetics all the time and this is how a diabetic wound begins to develop. A diabetic wound is an open sore usually under the ball of the foot. They can be difficult to treat, especially if they are infected. If an infection gets really bad, amputation of a toe or part of the foot may be a possibility. In fact, diabetics are 30 to 40 times more like to undergo a major amputation.

The most important thing a podiatrist can do is catch a peripheral neuropathy problem before it becomes bigger. Your podiatrist can debride, or shave down, calluses on the bottom of your feet. Calluses are common sites for diabetic wounds.

Constant rubbing from the inside of a shoe or rough surface can break the skin and lead to wounds. Your podiatrist can prescribe custom orthotics and make pads that can be used to reduce friction on the feet. If a foot exam reveals that you have peripheral neuropathy and you have not been diagnosed with diabetes, then your podiatrist will refer you to the right physician so you can be tested for diabetes and begin treatment, if needed. It is also important for diabetics who are over the age of 50 to have a test for peripheral artery disease, which occurs when there is a buildup of cholesterol and plaque in the arteries of the lower extremities, causing decreased blood flow to the legs and feet. This can lead to a poorly healing wound in your feet and increased risk of amputation.

Chapter 5

Foot Tips

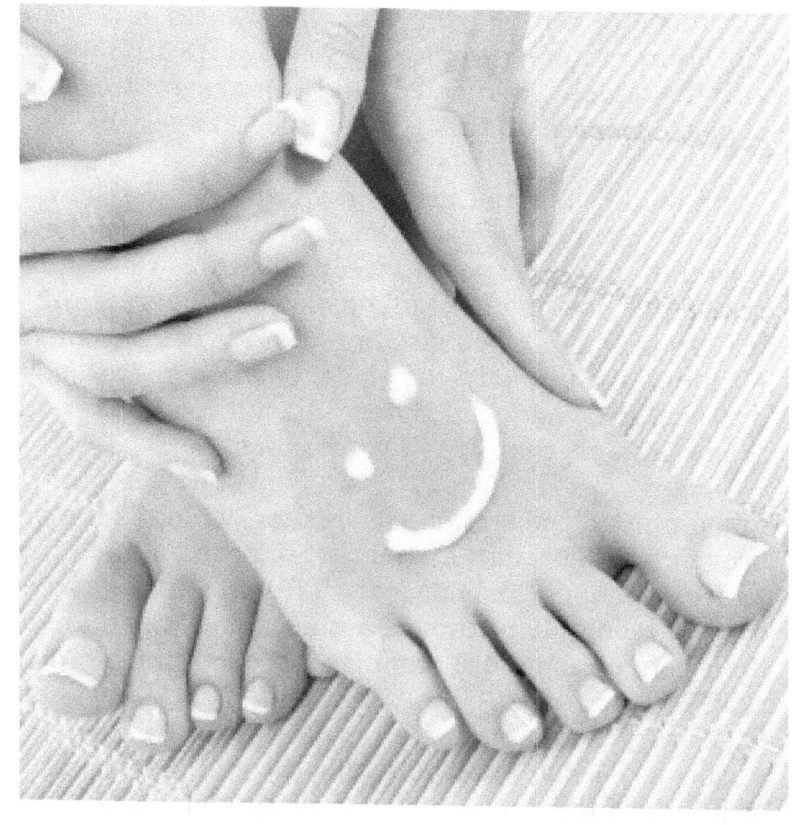

Do Rented Bowling Shoes Pose a Health Risk?

Published: *9-21-13*

I was recently interviewed by the editors of HGTV magazine for their September issue to comment in their section "How Bad is It ..." and to explain whether rented bowling shoes pose a health risk.

I have commented vigorously throughout my blogs, Facebook and Twitter about the importance of sterilizing shoes to prevent fungal infections of the feet and toenails, and was asked the question, "What may be lurking inside those leather lace-up bowling shoes that dozens, if not hundreds, of people have worn?"

Rented bowling shoes can be a host to several microorganisms including fungus, bacteria and the virus that causes warts. Although the likelihood of getting a virus such as warts or a bacterial infection of the foot from rented bowling shoes is low, if you have a blister or open sore and the shoes are infected, and you are not wearing socks, then it is possible to pick up this type of infection very easily.

Fungus likes a moist, dark environment, so if bowling shoes are damp from sweat and have an odor, don't be shy, ask for another pair. It would always be best to wear moisture-wicking socks that are copper infused or have nano bamboo charcoal fibers. Both of these materials help to promote blood circulation and restrain microbial growth. Although it's unlikely your local bowling alley is using a UV light to disinfect the insides of shoes, this is the most effective method of killing the organisms that live in your shoes.

I recommend the sterishoe sanitizer, which is the only product clinically proven to kill up to 99.9 percent of problematic microorganisms that cause onychomycosis or toenail fungus, athlete's foot and offensive shoe odor. I recommend this as a must for all my diabetic patients as part of their general foot care regimen since foot infections are a major health risk.

At the very least, a bowling alley should incorporate an antifungal spray or powder in-between use of their rented shoes. The best fungicidal, sanitizing deodorant spray for your shoes is Mycomist, which incorporates the active ingredients chlorophyll, formalin, and benzalkonium chloride. Formalin is a proven disinfectant and fumigant with penetrating power. Benzalkonium chloride is an all-purpose antibacterial agent, and is a good disinfectant for fungi. It is useful in sterile storage, and as a detergent as well as a germicide. Chlorophyll is used effectively for deodorization.

Other good choices are Lotrimine AF liquid spray and Zeasorb AF powder. Without sterilizing a shoe properly, the chance for fungal infections rises. A fungal infection of the skin is easier to clear than one of the nails. The disease, characterized by a change in a toenail's color, is often considered nothing more than a mere blemish. Left untreated, however, it can present serious problems and lead to painful thickened toenails that can take years to treat.

Also referred to as onychomycosis, fungal nails are infections underneath the surface of the nail, which penetrate the nail. Fungal nail infections are often accompanied by a secondary bacterial and/or yeast infection in or about the nail plate, which ultimately can lead to difficulty and pain when walking or running. Symptoms may include discoloration, brittleness, loosening, thickening or crumbling of the nail. A group of fungi, called dermophytes, easily attack the nail and thrive on keratin, the nail's protein substance.

In some cases, when these tiny organisms take hold, the nail may become thicker, yellowish-brown or darker in color, and foul smelling. Debris may collect beneath the nail plate, white marks may frequently appear on the nail plate, and the infection is capable of spreading to other toenails, the skin, or even the fingernails. I always recommend that people purchase their own bowling shoes if they plan on playing frequently.

The bottom line is that sterilization of bowling shoes in-between customers is important. If your bowling alley is not doing this, bring along some anti-fungal spray such as Lotrimine AF liquid spray and spray them yourself. Remember to always wear a good pair of anti-microbial socks lined with copper or bamboo fibers. And finally, if you plan to play often or are in a league, invest in a pair of good bowling shoes that fit properly and you won't have to worry!

At Odds: Smoking and Foot Surgery

Published: 8-3-13

By now, most of us have learned that smoking is very bad for our health. The facts about smoking are downright scary. Smoking has been linked to cancer, heart disease, stroke and lung diseases including emphysema, bronchitis and chronic airway obstruction.

With that said, smoking is the most preventable cause of death. Each year in the United States, smoking causes one out of every five deaths. This is more than 440,000 deaths a year. Smoking is also a very costly habit. Each year, diseases caused by smoking result in 96 billion in health care costs. Much of this money is paid by taxpayers through publicly funded health programs.

If the above is not enough to make you think twice about smoking, here is another fact for you: smoking can lead to poor healing after foot surgery. Research has shown that smoking has a negative effect on bone, skin and wound healing. Tobacco smoke has more than 7,000 chemicals and hundreds of these chemicals act like poison during healing. Nicotine and carbon monoxide are two chemicals in cigarette smoke that decrease healing after surgery. Nicotine narrows blood vessels resulting in decreased blood flow and oxygen. Adequate blood flow and oxygen is essential for any type of foot surgery because of the many tendons and bones in the feet-more than any other part of the body.

In fact, your podiatrist cannot even perform surgery if vascular testing shows that you do not have good blood flow to your feet. Nicotine also decreases osteoblast activity. Osteoblasts are the building cells of bones and are critical in bone healing after foot surgery. Carbon monoxide, like nicotine, also plays a role in limiting oxygen to the tissues. Smoking is also linked to an increased risk for infection after surgery.

Neutrophils are white blood cells that help the body fight off bacteria. Neutrophils kill bacteria by using oxygen. As you know now, smoking makes it difficult for oxygen to be used by the body. If neutrophils cannot do their job, bacteria are able to get into the operation sites and can cause much damage.

If you are thinking about getting a bunion or hammer toe fixed, you should seriously think about quitting smoking. Studies have shown that quitting smoking four to six weeks before surgery can improve surgical healing and give you a better outcome. Sometimes we have no control over life events and if you are in an accident you will not have time to quit smoking before a surgeon operates. In times like these, you want to have the advantage of having maximum blood flow and oxygen delivery. This just is not possible if you are a smoker.

If you are a diabetic, each cigarette you smoke is even more deadly. Diabetics already have an increased risk of poor healing and decreased blood flow. Sometimes foot surgery is necessary in diabetics and cigarette smokers are almost guaranteed to have a negative outcome.

Now that you know more facts, it's time to make a healthier life choice. Nobody said quitting smoking was easy, but as the facts show, your life depends on it.

If you are interested in fixing your foot deformities, stop smoking and see your podiatrist.

Pedicure Tips for the Summer and Beyond

Published: 7-13-13

Getting a pedicure is an enjoyable pastime, especially during the summer. Even if you get regular podiatric care, it feels good to look down and see perfectly polished toes and feel pampered for an hour or so. Pedicures may seem harmless, but there are reasons to be concerned. Every year, many people get hurt while getting a pedicure. Some people even get serious bacterial infections that began with a small pedicure injury.

Your podiatrist may not polish your toes, but he will definitely keep your feet and toenails looking healthy all year round. If you still feel like you need to go to the salon or spa, at least be safe. Use these tips to keep your toes pretty and healthy:

1. Know about your health.
If you are going to get a pedicure, you should definitely know as much as you can about your feet and overall health. Are you a diabetic? Do you have poor circulation? Do you take long to heal? Are you on blood thinners? These are very important things to consider. Diabetics need to be extremely careful. In fact, it may be best for diabetics to avoid getting pedicures from someone who is not a medical professional. If you have serious health conditions, ask your podiatrist and doctor if it is OK for you to even get a pedicure. You do not have to tell your pedicurist your whole medical history, but let them know that you have health concerns and infection risks so that they can be extremely careful with your feet. A careless nick from a pedicurist can lead to a long healing sore in some people.

2. Know as much as possible about your pedicurist and salon.
Be sure that your pedicurist is licensed by the state. The license should be displayed so you can see it. Check out the salon when you arrive. Is it clean? Does your pedicurist wash her hands before touching you? Does your pedicurist wear gloves? Does the foot bath have a disposable liner? You should ask how often the salon cleans their foot bath and changes the filter if they don't use disposable liners. Also, look at the tools that your pedicurist uses. Are they clean? Does the pedicurist sterilize them in an autoclave and un-wrap them in front of you? These are all important questions that you need to know. If the salon has an issue answering your questions, it is okay to decline service and go to a place where you feel more comfortable. Look for a Medi-Spa that is supervised by medical professionals.

3. Remember a pedicurist is not a podiatrist.
Pedicurists are very skilled and know how to make your toes pretty, but, remember, they are not medical professionals. It may be tempting to let a pedicurist remove a corn, callus or part of a toenail, but just say no. A pedicurist should never use a scalpel on your foot. Even if you trust them and they seem to know what they are doing, the risks are too great.

4. Learn to do it yourself.
If you see a podiatrist regularly, you will notice that over time your feet and toenails will look better. Once your toenails become more manageable, it may be possible for you to paint your own toenails. But remember to use nail polishes that don't contain toxic ingredients and are enriched with naturally-occurring elements like tea-tree oil, garlic bulb extract, wheat protein and Vitamins C and E.

Make sure you remove polish regularly to check the health of your toenails. If you notice a change in the color or thickness of your nails, make an appointment with your podiatrist. Fungal infections of your nails can spread quickly and become a painful condition if not treated early. They also take months to grow out.

Sometimes beauty is painful, but this does not have to be the case for your feet. Be smart and keep your feet looking their best this summer.

Feet Can Hold Clues to Heart Health

Published: 4-21-12

If you're wondering about the health of your heart, try looking at your feet. The lowly, stepped-on, shoe-squished foot could very well hold clues about the state of your coronary arteries.

If your feet show signs of poor circulation, or peripheral arterial disease, your heart could be suffering as well.

I regularly check patients for the subtle signs that could indicate peripheral arterial disease.

Approximately 9 million Americans over the age of 50 are living with peripheral arterial disease that affects their legs and raises their risk of having a heart attack. Unfortunately, many people with the disease do not even know they have it.

Peripheral arterial disease occurs when arteries in the legs become narrowed or clogged with fatty deposits, reducing blood flow to the legs. This can result in leg muscle pain when walking, disability, amputation and poor quality of life.

If you have blocked arteries somewhere in the body, you are likely to have them elsewhere. Thus, peripheral arterial disease is a red flag that other arteries, including those in the heart, are likely affected. This increases the risk of heart disease, heart attack and even death.

Peripheral arterial disease is a silent disease, causing no immediately recognizable symptoms. Often, people think the symptoms are just part of the aging process. This includes a loss of hair on the feet.

Fatigue, heaviness, tiredness or cramping in the leg muscles (calf, thigh or buttocks) that occurs during activity such as walking and then goes away with rest is also an indication of poor circulation.

Sometimes my patients will have toe or foot pain when they are resting that often disturbs their sleep. Many of my patients think this leg and foot discomfort is just part of "getting older," but it could indicate more serious problems.

Different pulses, very cold feet or a change in color also could indicate a circulation problem.

If I see any signs of peripheral arterial disease, I recommend a simple, non-invasive test called an ankle-brachial index. It compares the blood pressure in the ankles to the blood pressure in the arms.

Everyone over the age of 50 is at risk for peripheral arterial disease, and their risk increases if they have diabetes, high blood pressure, high cholesterol or if they are African- American.

In my practice, I recommend all patients who are over the age of 50 have an ankle-brachial index test done if they have diabetes and at least one other risk factor such as a history of smoking, abnormal cholesterol or high blood pressure.

Diabetics that have skin wounds or ulcers on their feet or toes, that are slow to heal, or that do not heal for 8 to 12 weeks, are good indicators of poor circulation. If a patient is over the age of 70, then I recommend they get tested even if they don't have any risk factors.

If you fit into any of the above groups, talk to your health care provider about being tested for peripheral arterial disease. Through early detection and proper treatment, we can reduce the devastating consequences of peripheral arterial disease and improve the nation's cardiovascular health.

Foot Tips for Summer Picnics

Published: *7-2-11*

Dust off your frisbee and find the cooler: It's time to head for a backyard cookout or a picnic in the park. This is what you dreamed about all through those cold, crummy winter months. But, eager as you are to get out there and play some tag football, or to hit the hammock with a burger clutched in each fist, you need to be warned. Here are some foot tips for a safer summer picnic:

- See a foot and ankle surgeon within 24 hours for a puncture wound. Why? These injuries can embed unsterile foreign objects deep inside the foot. A puncture wound must be cleaned properly and monitored as it heals. This will help to avoid complications such as tissue and bone infections or damage to tendons and muscles in the foot.

- Beware of charcoal or a stray "hot" coal on the ground. Why? They can be dangerous in the bag or out. Some bags may weigh 10 pounds or more, and that force increases when they drop on your bare foot. Toe and nail injuries can lead to permanently deformed toenails that become susceptible to fungus. People can also suffer serious burns from accidentally stepping on stray campfire coals or fireworks. That stray sparkler on the ground can also cause a nasty burn if stepped on with a bare foot.

- Make sure you've been vaccinated against tetanus. Experts recommend teens and adults get a booster shot every 10 years. Why? Cuts and puncture wounds from sharp objects can lead to infections and illnesses such as tetanus. If your summer just wouldn't be the same without kicking off your shoes, you can still stay safe. Just watch where you walk!

- Watch out for holes covered by grass! Why? The jarring that occurs when a person takes a step and then meets air, not solid ground, and subsequently hits hard after just falling a few inches can cause a great deal of damage to the foot, including breaks and fractures.

- Watch out for that cool breeze and falling asleep on that pretty colored blanket. Why? Feet get sunburned, too, and rare but deadly skin cancers can develop on the feet. Apply sunscreen to the tops and bottoms of your feet, not just your legs.

- Inspect your feet and your children's feet on a routine basis for skin problems such as warts, calluses, ingrown toenails and suspicious moles, spots or freckles. Why? The earlier a skin condition is detected, the easier it is for your foot and ankle surgeon to treat it.

- Wear slides or sandals around swimming pools, locker rooms and beaches. Why? Wearing this foot protection can help you avoid cuts and abrasions from rough anti-slip surfaces and sharp objects hidden beneath sandy beaches, and prevent contact with bacteria and viruses that can cause athlete's foot, plantar warts and other problems.

- Use common sense with going barefoot. Why? Every year, people lose toes while mowing the lawn barefoot. People with diabetes should never go barefoot, even indoors, because their nervous system may not "feel" an injury and their circulatory system will struggle to heal breaks in the skin. So you see, don't just let the ants or mosquitoes ruin your picnic. Be careful and protect your feet.

Travel Tips for Deep Leg Thrombosis

Published: *4-16-11*

Spring has sprung and the travel season has begun! It's time to pack your bags and head off to your favorite destination. But while you're riding in the car or travelling by plane, remember to stretch those legs to help prevent a serious condition known as deep vein thrombosis.

Deep vein thrombosis is a condition in which a blood clot, a blockage, forms in a vein located deep within the leg.

These clots most commonly occur in the veins of the leg, but can also develop in other parts of the body.

If the clot breaks loose and travels through the bloodstream, it can lodge in the lung. This blockage in the lung, called a pulmonary embolism, can make it difficult to breathe and may even cause death.

Some people are more at risk than others for developing deep vein thrombosis. Risk factors include varicose veins, blood clotting disorders, pregnancy or recent childbirth, obesity, tobacco use and heart disease.

People over 40 years old, those who have had recent surgery, or those who are immobile through inactivity or wearing a cast are also more at risk for deep vein thrombosis. People with deep vein thrombosis in the leg may have either no warning signs or their symptoms can be very vague.

If any of the following warning signs or symptoms are present, it is important to make an appointment for an evaluation.

- Swelling in the leg
- Pain in the calf or thigh
- Warmth and redness of the leg

If you are at risk for deep vein thrombosis and plan on taking a long trip this season, follow these tips to reduce the likelihood of developing a blood clot:

- Exercise legs every two to three hours to get the blood flowing back to the heart. Walk up and down the aisle of a plane or train, rotate ankles while sitting and take regular breaks on road trips.
- Stay hydrated by drinking plenty of fluids and avoid caffeine and alcohol.
- Consider wearing compression stockings.

Fit shoes in the afternoon and compression stockings in the morning. That's the simple but effective rule that works. For diabetics, usually we suggest 15 to 20 mmHg compression for those with edema and 10 to 15 mmHg for those without. For anything higher than 20mmHg compression, patients should be custom measured by a physician, especially if they have peripheral arterial disease.

New Year's Resolution Safety Tips at the Gym

Published: *1-15-11*

Don't forget to keep your feet in tip-top shape while following through with your resolutions to get fit.

Let me offer some tips for foot safety while at the gym.

- **Start new workouts gradually.**

Increase your stamina and the length of your workouts gradually to avoid overuse injuries such as stress fractures or tendon strains and sprains.

Stretching your muscles before and after workouts also helps prevent these types of injuries. If you do feel you've sprained your ankle, be sure to seek treatment right away.

Untreated or repeated ankle sprains may lead to chronic ankle instability, a condition that causes persistent pain and a "giving way" of the ankle.

- **Wear the right shoes and socks.**

Wear well-fitting athletic shoes designed for the exercise or sport.

Shoes that don't support the arch of the foot and provide cushion for the heel can cause heel pain, called plantar fasciitis.

Shoes that are too small can also cause a neuroma, or a thickening of the nerve tissue, in the foot and may require injections, medication or physical therapy.

Wearing cotton or non-slip socks is also key to help avoid painful blisters, which can become infected and cause more serious issues.

New fibers in socks such as copper and bamboo help to whisk away moisture and are naturally anti-microbial and antifungal.

The recently trapped Chilean coal miners were given copper socks to keep their feet dry and help protect against fungus.

- **Use good technique.**

Improper exercise techniques can result in injury to the tendons or ligaments in your feet and ankles.

Incorrect posture or misuse of exercise equipment can cause decreased stabilization in the foot and ankle, leading to joint sprains and muscle strains.

- **Protect yourself from bacteria.**

Sweaty shoes, public showers, exercise equipment and the pool deck at the gym are breeding grounds for fungus, viruses and bacteria, including drug-resistant strains like methicillin resistant Staphylococcus aureus, which has become increasingly more common.

Never go barefoot while in public areas. Water shoes can provide a great barrier between your feet and the wet surfaces.

It's also best to cover cuts and cracks in the skin or ingrown toenails, since these minor tears in the skin's surface can act as entry points for bacteria.

If you have a cut or scrape that becomes red or swollen and is not healing in a timely manner, don't hesitate to see a foot and ankle surgeon for an examination.

Above all, it's important to listen to your body. If you experience an injury or have pain, call your podiatrist for an evaluation.

Five Tips for Healthy Holiday Feet

Published: *12-18-10*

Don't let sore, achy feet ruin your holiday season. Here are five tips for healthy holiday feet.

If the shoe fits, wear it

When hitting the dance floor or the shopping malls during the holiday season, don't compromise comfort and safety when picking the right shoes to wear.

Narrow shoes, overly high heels or shoes that aren't worn very often can irritate feet and lead to blisters, calluses, swelling and even severe ankle injuries.

To ward off problems, choose a shoe that has a low heel and fits your foot in length, width and depth while you are standing.

Remember my three P's of shoe selection: Be proactive, protective and preventive with your selection of appropriate shoes for the occasion.

Don't overindulge in holiday cheer

Did you know your feet can feel the effects of too much holiday cheer?

Certain foods and beverages high in purines, such as shellfish, red meat, red wine and beer can trigger extremely painful gout attacks, a condition when uric acid builds up and crystallizes in and around your joints.

Oftentimes, it's the big toe that is affected first since the toe is the coolest part of the body and uric acid is sensitive to temperature changes.

Be pedicure-safety conscious

Before you head for your holiday pedicure, remember nail salons can be a breeding ground for bacteria.

To reduce your risk of infection, choose a salon that follows proper sanitation practices. Consider purchasing your own pedicure instruments to bring along to your appointment.

Watch for ice and snow

Holiday winter wonderlands can be beautiful and dangerous. Use caution when traveling outdoors. Watch for ice or snow patches along your trail.

The ankle joint can be more vulnerable to serious injury from falling on ice.

Ice accelerates the fall and often causes more severe trauma, because the foot can move in any direction after it slips.

Consider purchasing traction grips for your shoes. You can find these at sporting goods stores and they can be used on dress or athletic shoes.

If you do experience a fall, take a break from activities until you can be seen by a foot and ankle surgeon.

Use R.I.C.E. therapy (rest, ice, compression and elevation) to help reduce the pain and control swelling around the injury.

"Listen" to your feet

Don't let foot pain ruin your holiday fun; inspect your feet regularly for any evidence of ingrown toenails, bruising, swelling, blisters, dry skin or calluses.

If you notice any pain, swelling or signs of problems, make an appointment with your foot and ankle surgeon.

Often, especially for diabetics, what may seem like a simple issue can turn into a larger problem if medical care is delayed.

If you are suffering from foot pain or have concerns about your foot health, call your podiatrist for an evaluation.

Seven Myths About Footcare

Published: 9-18-10

"Don't cross your eyes, they'll stay that way!"

Old wives' tales and myths like this are fun to laugh at. We believed them as children.

"Step on a crack and you'll break your mother's back."

But there are other myths that are no laughing matter, especially when they involve your health.

From bunions to broken toes, I have heard it all. Let me share seven myths about foot care and the realities behind them that I have heard from patients.

Myth: Cutting a notch, a V, in a toenail will relieve the pain of ingrown toenails.

Reality: When a toenail is ingrown, the nail curves downward and grows into the skin. Cutting a V in the toenail does not affect its growth. New nail growth will continue to curve downward.

Cutting a V may actually cause more problems and can be painful in many cases.

Myth: My foot or ankle can't be broken if I can walk on it.

Reality: It's entirely possible to walk on a foot or ankle with a broken bone. It depends on your threshold for pain, as well as the severity of the injury. But it's not a smart idea. Walking with a broken bone can cause further damage. It is crucial to stay off an injured foot until diagnosis by a foot and ankle surgeon. Until then, apply ice and elevate the foot to reduce pain.

Myth: Shoes cause bunions.

Reality: Bunions are most often caused by an inherited faulty mechanical structure of the foot. It is not the bunion itself that is inherited, but certain foot types that make a person prone to developing a bunion. While wearing shoes that crowd the toes together can, over time, make bunions more painful, shoes themselves do not cause bunions. Although some treatments can ease the pain of bunions, only surgery can correct the deformity.

Myth: A doctor can't fix a broken toe.

Reality: Nineteen of the 26 bones in the foot are toe bones. There are things we can do to make a broken toe heal better and prevent problems later on, like arthritis or toe deformities. Broken toes that aren't treated correctly can also make walking and wearing shoes difficult. A foot and ankle surgeon will X-ray the toe to learn more about the fracture. If the broken toe is out of alignment, the surgeon may have to insert a pin, screw or plate to reposition the bone.

Myth: Corns Have Roots

Reality: A corn is a small build-up of skin caused by friction. Many corns result from a hammertoe deformity, where the toe knuckle rubs against the shoe. The only way to eliminate these corns is to surgically correct the hammertoe condition. Unlike a callus, a corn has a central core of hard material, but corns do not have roots. Attempting to cut off a corn or applying medicated corn pads can lead to serious infection or even amputation. A foot and ankle surgeon can safely evaluate and treat corns and the conditions contributing to them.

Myth: Warts can be "suffocated" with duct tape or salve.

Reality: While warts may be living viruses, they cannot be suffocated. Warts can appear anywhere on the skin, but technically only those on the sole of the foot are properly called plantar warts. Your podiatric physician can prescribe and supervise your use of a safe and appropriate wart-removal preparation. Removal of warts may also be done through a simple surgical procedure performed under local anesthesia. People with diabetes or circulatory, immunological or neurological problems should be especially careful with the treatment of their warts and seek professional care at all times.

Myth: Heel spurs are "calcium deposits."

Reality: A heel spur is most often the result of stress on the muscles and fascia of the foot. This stress may form a spur on the bottom of the heel. While many spurs are painless, others may produce chronic pain. Based on the condition and the chronic nature of the disease, your podiatrist may suggest orthotics and stretching exercises for pain relief. New conservative treatments such as blood platelet injection or Shockwave therapy used by professional athletes have shown great results.

Heel surgery, as a last resort, can provide relief of pain and restore mobility in many cases. The type of procedure is based on examination and usually consists of plantar fascia release, with or without heel spur excision. There have been various modifications and surgical enhancements regarding surgery of the heel.

Your podiatric physician will determine which method is best suited for you.

Healthy Feet Make the Best Dancing Feet

Published: 3-1-10

If you plan to be light on your feet at the Feb. 27 Day of Dance in Findlay, remember to be careful. Amateur and professional dancers can suffer foot injuries that can stop the show, as witnessed on the popular television show "Dancing with the Stars." More than 50 percent of dance injuries occur in the foot and ankle.

The severity of the damage is determined by your age, strength, flexibility and the type of shoes worn when dancing. The most common types of problems are overuse injuries, which occur due to the repetitive movements in dance.

There are several other common types of injuries related to dancing. Stress fractures, or hairline breaks in the bone, can occur from repeated jumping and landing. Special taping techniques performed by a podiatrist can help prevent these types of injuries.

Foot neuromas, also known as the thickening or irritation of nerves in the ball of the foot, result from repetitive pivoting. Pressure from poorly fitting shoes or an abnormal bone structure can also lead to this condition.

Symptoms may include sensations of thickness, burning, numbness, tingling, or pain in the ball of the foot. Shin splints, or pain and swelling in the front of the lower legs, can be aggravated by recurring activities.

The problem is usually related to a collapsing arch but may be caused by a muscle imbalance between opposing muscle groups in the leg.

Proper stretching before and after exercise and sports, corrective shoes, or orthotics, also known as corrective shoe inserts, can help prevent shin splints.

Tendonitis, or inflammation of the tendons in the foot, can result from overexertion.

A common overuse injury, Achilles tendonitis, often begins with mild pain after exercise or running that gradually worsens. Morning tenderness about 1.5 inches above the point where the Achilles tendon is attached to the heel bone is common.

Corns, calluses or blisters are all painful skin irritations resulting from repeated rubbing of the skin on the feet.

Special over-the-counter, non-medicated, donut-shaped foam pads can be worn to relieve the pressure and discomfort.

Since dancing is repetitive and hard on the lower extremities, how can dancers protect their feet and ankles at the 'Day of Dance' and the days afterward?

The best defense is prevention. Dancers should wear shoes that properly support their feet and ankles.

A properly fitted and supportive shoe, combined with an accommodative shoe insert, can put your feet in balance and improve your body alignment.

In addition, dancers should remember their individual skill level when performing dance moves. Don't overdo it!

If an injury does occur, prompt medical attention by a foot and ankle surgeon can make all the difference in a proper rehabilitation.

Most dance injuries can be treated with conservative care as long as they are addressed early and not ignored.

Many people try to ignore foot pain if they can walk on the foot, but remember that it is possible to walk on a seriously injured foot. If left untreated, even common injuries may require surgical intervention to ensure proper healing.

If you are suffering from foot or ankle pain, contact your podiatrist for an assessment.

Beach Barefoot Safety Tips

Published: 6-6-09

As families hit the beach this summer, I'd like to share safety tips that will help your feet stay healthy and pain-free. Everyone should keep these items in their beach bag:

- Antibacterial cream or ointment for cuts or wounds.
- Bandages that are self-adherent and waterproof.
- Non-refrigerant cold and compression packs.
- Good sunscreen or lotion, SPF 30 or higher.

A day at the beach doesn't have to mean a day in the emergency room, so keep these tips in mind.

As always, any injury that doesn't resolve within a few days should be examined by a foot and ankle surgeon.

Wear shoes to protect your feet from sea shells, broken glass and other sharp objects. If you wear flip flops, try gel toe spreaders. They wrap around the thong to reduce friction and add comfort in flip-flops and sandals.

Wear a diver's sock or shoe to protect your feet in the water.

Don't go in the water if your skin gets cut, since bacteria in oceans and lakes can cause infections. Use antibacterial cream or ointment, followed by a waterproof, self-adherent bandage. To avoid complications, see a foot and ankle surgeon for treatment within 24 hours.

Jellyfish can sting you in the water or on the beach, so be careful! If a jellyfish's tentacles stick to your foot or ankle, remove them, but protect your hands from getting stung. Vinegar, meat tenderizer, baking soda or soaking your foot in a bath can reduce pain and swelling.

Most jellyfish stings heal within a few days. If yours doesn't, seek medical treatment.

Feet get sunburned, too. Apply sunscreen to the tops and bottoms of your feet. Already been sunburned? Use a nourishing lotion with vitamin E and aloe vera to soothe your skin. Sand, sidewalks and paved surfaces get hot in the summer sun. Wear shoes to protect your soles from getting burned, especially if you have diabetes.

Walking, jogging and playing sports on soft, uneven surfaces like sand can lead to arch pain, heel pain, ankle sprains and other injuries. Athletic shoes provide the heel cushioning and arch support that flip-flops and sandals lack.

If injuries occur use rest, ice, compression and elevation to ease pain and swelling.

Keep a travel-size ice compression pack in your beach bag that doesn't require refrigeration. It's a must when on-the-spot cold compression is needed.

Americans with diabetes face serious foot safety risks at the beach. Diabetes causes poor blood circulation and numbness in the feet, meaning they might not feel pain from a cut, puncture wound or burn.

Any type of skin break on a diabetic foot has the potential to get infected and ulcerate if it isn't noticed right away.

Diabetics should always wear shoes to the beach and remove them regularly to check for foreign objects like sand and shells that can cause sores, ulcers or infections.

Eliminate Foot Pain to Lose Weight

Published: *4-18-09*

Excess weight can cause foot pain. However, it's tough to lose weight when your feet hurt.

Being overweight or obese changes the way your foot functions. Force on your foot increases, your steps are shorter, your feet angle out more and flattening of the foot increases.

Studies have shown that overweight patients experience more heel pain, tendonitis, arthritis, ball-of-foot pain, fractures and sprains in their feet and ankles than patients at a normal weight.

So what do you do if foot pain from excess weight prevents you from exercising?

Reducing foot pain will allow you to exercise in comfort, helping you lose weight safely and improving your health.

Foot orthotics can minimize abnormal force on the feet and are often used to treat and prevent foot problems for those carrying excess weight and/or trying to lose weight.

A firm, controlling foot orthotic can support the forces caused by extra weight and provide shock absorption to decrease the stress on your joints and prevent arthritis.

The best orthotics are those that conform closely to the arch of the foot.

Though prefabricated orthotics are available, they often do not provide enough support to adequately relieve pain.

People carrying excess weight are more likely to need custom orthotics for the best pain relief.

Other treatments for foot pain caused by excess weight include stretching, strengthening and anti-inflammatory measures.

If you are starting a weight loss program, be sure to talk to your primary care physician, a registered dietician, and personal trainer or physical therapist to create the best exercise program for your needs.

Taking a Vacation? Make it Easy on your Feet!

Published: *5-9-09*

Although rest and relaxation are the goals for most vacations, they usually involve a lot of walking. Unfortunately, a lot of walking usually involves sore feet. Walking is a great exercise and one of the most reliable forms of transportation. However, if your feet aren't in the best shape or you don't have the right shoes, too much walking can cause foot problems. Good foot care is essential if you plan to subject your feet to long periods of walking.

Here are some simple foot care tips:

- Wear thick, absorbent socks. Try acrylic instead of cotton.
- Dry feet thoroughly after bathing, making sure to dry between your toes. Use powder before putting on shoes.
- Nails should be cut regularly, straight across the toe.
- Bunions, hammertoes or any other serious foot problems should be evaluated by a foot-and-ankle surgeon.

The right shoe is also important to healthy walking. The ideal walking shoe is stable from side to side, well-cushioned, and will allow you to walk smoothly. While many running shoes will fit the bill, there are also shoes made specially for walking. Walking shoes tend to be slightly less cushioned and are not as bulky. They are also lighter than running shoes. Whether you choose a walking or running shoe, the shoes need to feel stable and comfortable. Warm-up exercises that are done before walking can help alleviate muscle stiffness or pulled muscles. Loosening up the thigh muscles and heel cords (in the Achilles and calf) before a walk is especially effective. If you're not used to long walks, start slowly and rest if your feet start to hurt.

Above all, have fun!

Chapter 6

General Foot Injuries

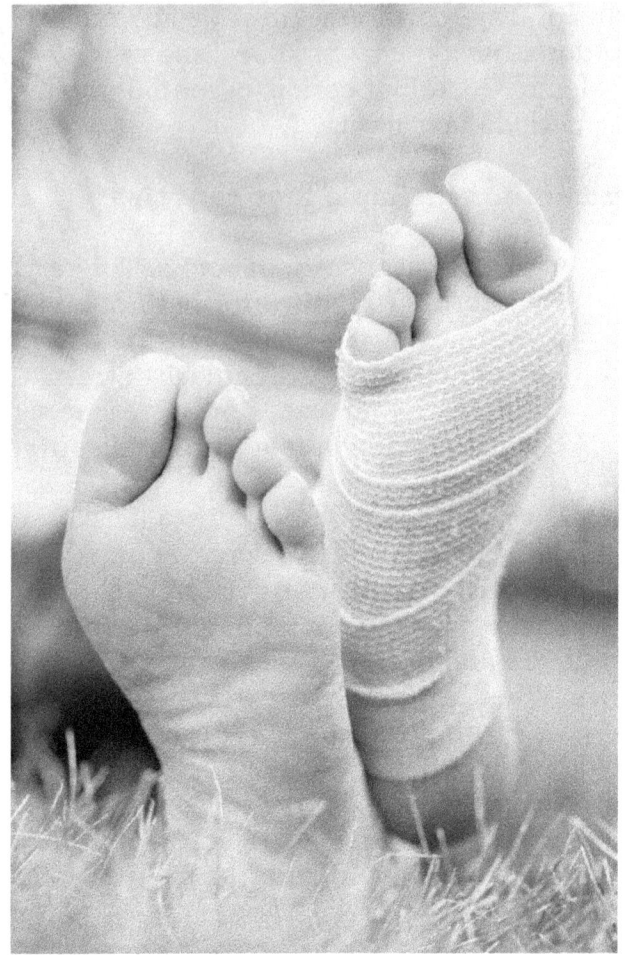

Fractures of the Body can Cause Foot Damage

Published: 9-7-13

I've talked in previous articles about fractures of the foot and what causes them and how to treat them. But my patients often ask me if I fracture or injure another part of my body, such as my back, legs or hip, can this be of concern for damage to my feet? Fractures or injuries in other parts of the body can definitely affect the nerves in the foot and cause vascular problems.

Fractures happen when there's more force applied to the bone than the bone can absorb. These breaks in bones can occur from falls, trauma or a direct blow. With children heading back to school, sports related fractures are a common occurrence.

Fractures are not limited, though, to trauma or overuse injuries. Over time, a person with osteoporosis may also experience stress fractures, especially in their back.

Any type of fracture can cause an injury to the nerves and develop into a vascular problem. For the lower extremity, the two major nerves that one is primarily concerned with after a traumatic injury are the tibial nerve and common peroneal nerve.

These two nerves originate from the sciatic nerve. The sciatic nerve is the big nerve running from the lower back, through the buttocks, and down to the lower limbs. If the sciatic nerve is injured, symptoms are pain, weakness, tingling or numbness from the lower back to the lower leg. If the tibial nerve is injured at the leg below the knee level and above the ankle, the patient will experience a loss in motor function and sensory to the calf muscles and the sole of the foot. If the tibial nerve injury is below or at the ankle level, the patient will lose the ability to move the foot down (plantar flexion), rotate the foot (inversion), curl the toe up (flexion) and, of course, sensory loss at the sole of the foot as well.

The peroneal nerve is a branch of the sciatic nerve, which supplies movement and sensation to the lower leg, foot and toes. Common peroneal nerve dysfunction is a type of peripheral neuropathy; damage to nerves outside the brain or spinal cord. This condition can affect people of any age.

If the common peroneal nerve is injured, the patient will experience a decrease in sensation, numbness or tingling on the top of the foot or the outer part of the upper or lower leg, foot drop, "slapping" gait, dragging toes, and weakness of the ankles or feet.

Dysfunction of a single nerve, such as the common peroneal nerve, is called a mononeuropathy. Mononeuropathy means the nerve damage occurred in one area. However, certain body-wide conditions may also cause single nerve injuries.

Damage to the nerve destroys the myelin sheath that covers the axon, a branch of the nerve cell. Or it may destroy the whole nerve cell. There is a loss of feeling, muscle control, muscle tone, and eventual loss of muscle mass because the nerves aren't stimulating the muscles.

Common causes of damage to the peroneal nerve include the following:
- Trauma or injury to the knee.

- Fracture of the fibula, a bone of the lower leg.
- Use of a tight plaster cast or other long-term constriction of the lower leg.
- Crossing the legs regularly.
- Regularly wearing high boots.
- Pressure to the knee from positions during deep sleep or coma.
- Injury during knee surgery or from being placed in an awkward position during anesthesia.

As mentioned above, a fracture can cause a vascular injury. Signs of vascular injury in the lower extremity are pulsatile bleeding, bruising, absent distal pulses, and a cold and pale limb. A doppler is commonly used to detect the pulses that couldn't be examined easily otherwise.

If you experience any of the symptoms above with or without a known injury, please make an appointment to visit your podiatrist to be evaluated for nerve dysfunction or injury.

Achilles Tendon Rupture Treatment

Published: *9-10-11*

You may have heard recently that "Jeopardy's" Alex Trebek ruptured his Achilles tendon while chasing a burglar down the hall at his San Francisco hotel.

On July 27, Trebek was using crutches before opening the final round of the National Geographic World Championship. He explained that a female burglar broke into his hotel room at 2:30 a.m. July 26, while staying at the downtown Marriott, when he and his wife were sleeping.

Awakened by the intruder, he chased her down the hallway, but his Achilles tendon ripped, causing him to fall and bruise his other leg in the process. He had surgery last week.

Rupturing or tearing of the Achilles tendon is a common condition. This typically occurs in an individual who sustains the rupture while playing sports or perhaps from tripping. There is a vigorous contraction of the muscle and the tendon tears.

The patient will often describe the sensation as someone or something has hit the back of the calf muscle. Pain is suddenly present and, although it is possible to walk, it is painful and the leg is weak.

While it is possible to treat this ruptured tendon without surgery, this is never ideal since the maximum strength of the muscle and tendon never returns. Surgical correction of the ruptured tendon is necessary.

The surgery is performed in order to regain the maximum strength of the Achilles, as well as the normal pushing-off strength of the foot.

There are two types of surgery to repair a ruptured Achilles tendon:

- In open surgery, the surgeon makes a single large incision in the back of the leg.
- In percutaneous surgery, the surgeon makes several small incisions rather than one large incision.

In both types of surgery, the surgeon sews the tendon back together through the incision(s).

Surgery may be delayed for about a week after the rupture to let the swelling go down.

After either type of surgery, you will likely wear a cast, walking boot or a similar device for six to 12 weeks.

At first, the cast or boot is positioned to keep the foot pointed downward as the tendon heals. The cast or boot is then adjusted gradually to put the foot in a neutral position, not pointing up or down.

Many health professionals recommend starting movement and weight-bearing exercises early, before the cast or boot comes off. Your total recovery time will probably be as long as six months. Walking and exercise are very important after the surgery and a careful physical therapy program will be required.

In general, both open and percutaneous surgeries are successful. More than 80 out of 100 people who have surgery for an Achilles tendon rupture are able to return to all the activities they did before the injury, including sports.

If you suspect you have an Achilles injury, make an appointment as soon as possible with a podiatrist.

Lawnmowers: Use Caution to Avoid Foot Injury

Published: 5-21-11

Lawn care season is back and I caution homeowners to protect their feet and the feet of those around them when using rotary-blade lawnmowers. Each year, about 25,000 Americans sustain injuries from power mowers, according to the U.S. Consumer Products Safety Commission.

Yet, each year I continue to see patients who have been hurt while operating a lawnmower barefoot or wearing flip-flops. While electric mowers seem more dangerous because there is electricity involved, people even suffer injuries from just using a manual push model.

Children younger than 14 and adults older than 44, are more likely to be injured from mowers than other people. Anyone who operates a lawnmower should take a few simple precautions to avoid injuries or accidents:

- Don't mow a wet lawn. Losing control from slipping on rain-soaked grass is the leading cause of foot injuries caused by power mowers.

- Before starting to mow, take a good look around your garden and search it for sticks, rocks, toys, or dog bones, as these can all damage your mower. In addition, hitting these objects can cause the mower to veer out of control and cause serious injury.

- Goggles or other eye protection should be worn to protect foreign objects like stones from coming in contact with the blades, being thrown up and striking your eyes.

- If your mower strikes a foreign object, turn it off immediately, disconnect the power supply, and make sure the blades have stopped rotating before checking for any damage.

- Wear heavy shoes or work boots when mowing. No sneakers or sandals! Flimsy footwear like flip-flops put your feet at the most risk for injury. Steel-toe cap boots are preferable.

- Don't let small children ride on the lap of an adult on a lawn tractor. Children can be severely injured by the blades when getting on or off the machine

- If you leave your lawnmower for any length of time, turn the engine off and remember to take the key with you.

- Mow across slopes instead of up or down them to avoid falling or injuring yourself.

- Mow by pushing the mower away from you. Never pull a running mower backwards.

- Never mow over gravel.

- Keep children away from the lawn when mowing.

- When operating a power mower, keep the clip bag attached to prevent projectile injuries.

- Use a mower with a release mechanism on the handle that automatically shuts it off when your hands let go.

- Don't smoke when using a gasoline mower. Keep all ignition sources away from the mower and the fuel supply.

- Buy a mower that has a residual current device fitted. Should you inadvertently cut through a cable, this will immediately cut off the electricity supply.

- Always clean a mower after you use it, store it in a safe place, and keep it well maintained.

If a mower accident does occur, immediate treatment is necessary to flush the wound thoroughly and apply antibiotics to prevent infection. While superficial wounds can be treated on an outpatient basis, more serious injuries usually require surgery to deep-clean the wound and close it, or to repair tendon damage.

Winter is Fall Season

Published: 1-28-10

Falls on icy surfaces are a major cause of ankle sprains and fractures. It's critical to seek prompt treatment to prevent further damage that can prolong recovery. For women, this winter's fashionable high-heeled boots put them at higher risk for slips, falls and injuries on ice and snow. These popular boots typically feature tall, spiked heels and narrow, pointed toes. Wearing high heels makes you more unstable when walking or standing on dry surfaces, let alone slippery ones like ice or snow.

Falls from high-heeled winter boots can lead to a number of injuries, depending on how a woman loses her balance. In any event, a stylish, low-heeled winter boot is a lot more fashionable than a cast and crutches. I recommend scuffing-up the soles of new boots or purchasing adhesive rubber soles to provide greater traction. The ankle joint is vulnerable to serious injury from hard falls on ice.

Ice accelerates the fall and often causes more severe trauma because the foot can go in any direction after slipping. In cases of less-severe fractures and sprains, it is possible to walk and mistakenly believe the injury doesn't require medical treatment.

Never assume the ability to walk means your ankle is not broken or badly sprained. Putting weight on an injured joint can worsen the problem and lead to chronic instability, joint pain and arthritis later in life. Some people may even fracture and sprain an ankle at the same time. Believe it or not, a bad sprain can mask a fracture. It is best to have an injured ankle evaluated as soon as possible for proper diagnosis and treatment. If you can't get to a foot and ankle surgeon or the emergency room right away, follow the RICE technique - Rest, Ice, Compression, and Elevation - until medical care is available. Even though the symptoms of ankle sprains and fractures are similar, fractures are associated with:

- Pain at the site of the fracture that can extend from the foot to the knee.
- Significant swelling.
- Blisters over the fracture site.
- Bruising soon after the injury.
- Bone protruding through the skin, also known as a compound fracture, which requires immediate attention.

Most ankle fractures and some sprains are treated by immobilizing the joint in a cast or splint to promote union and healing. However, surgery may be needed to repair fractures with significant mal-alignment to unite bone fragments and realign them properly. Newly designed surgical plates and screws allow repair of these injuries with less surgical trauma. With newer bone-fixation methods, smaller incisions minimize tissue damage and bleeding and accelerate the healing process.

If you injure your ankle in any way, schedule an appointment with your podiatrist. If you fall on an icy spot and hurt your ankle, seek medical attention immediately. This aids in early diagnosis and proper treatment of the ankle injury and reduces the risk of further damage to your foot or ankle.

Chapter 7

Heel Pain

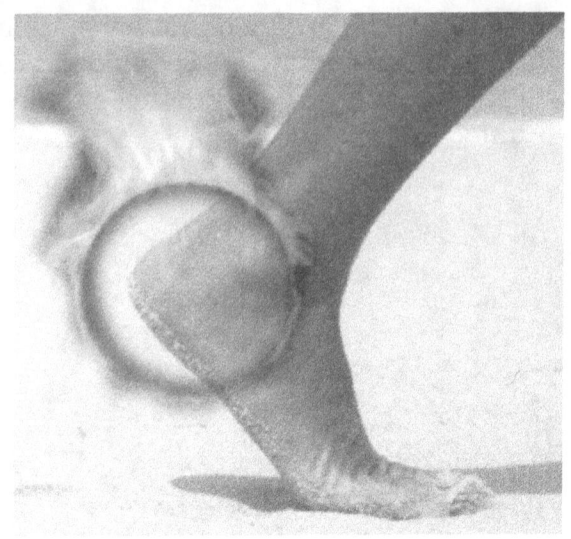

Victor Cruz: Not the Only One Affected by Heel Pain

Published: *11-2-13*

The only thing that could spoil all the positive energy of the National Football League season now is if one of your star players goes on the injured reserve list.

Victor Cruz, a New York Giants wide receiver, almost didn't make the opening games due to a heel injury on Aug. 18. Thankfully for Giants fans, he was able to play in the opening games, which meant his heel injury is almost completely behind him. Other players may not be so lucky though. Whether you are a pro-athlete or just a weekend sports enthusiast, some precautions should be taken to prevent you sitting on the sidelines.

Heel injuries are common in athletes, but it doesn't take a brutal contact sport like football to cause them. Plantar fasciitis is one of the most common foot pathologies I see in my practice. This disorder is responsible for more than 1 million patient visits every year in our country, so it is wise to know how to avoid this painful condition and how to treat it.

Pro-athletes are use to long and hard training sessions. But if you haven't trained or run in a while, it is best to start off slow and build momentum to avoid injury. Professional football players should know their own body limitations and make adjustments to the length and intensity of their training.

The plantar fascia is a thin band of tissue that is attached very closely to the skin on the bottom of your foot. If you stress it too much by exerting yourself too quickly, then micro-trauma to the tissue will result. Repetitive micro-trauma will lead to painful inflammation and you will develop heel pain that is most noticeable when you take your first step after getting out of bed in the morning. Always stretch before your workouts and make sure you are not taking on more than your body can handle.

Also known as heel spur syndrome, the condition is often successfully treated with conservative measures, such as anti-inflammatory medications, ice packs, stretching exercises and splints, custom orthotic devices, and physical therapy. Please consult your physician before taking any medications, though.

In persistent cases, autologous platelet concentrate — an injection into the plantar fascia using your own platelets, the healing trigger factor of blood — or extracorporeal shock wave treatment may be used to treat the heel pain. Many pro athletes have used these conservative approaches successfully to get back in the game without surgical intervention.

Faulty running shoes are another common cause of plantar fasciitis. You should make sure you are in an athletic shoe that is designed for the contours of your feet and the sport you are playing. You should also make sure that you are replacing your athletic shoes on a regular basis. The lifespan of your athletic shoe will be determined by the frequency of your sports activity. If you run or play sports daily, you may need to replace your shoes every six months or sooner. Your shoes may not show signs of wear, but the internal support in the arch and heel will not support your foot properly anymore and ultimately put stress on your feet that will cause damage. Replacing your shoes promptly at the first signs of foot pain may actually help you avoid a serious injury. Professional certified shoe fitters can match a specific running/athletic shoe to a certain foot type. A podiatrist with an interest in sports medicine could help you devise a running plan that would avoid this common foot disorder.

Lastly, avoid running on uneven surfaces and concrete. Your foot goes through a natural progression of very specific movements from when your heel first strikes the ground to when your toes leave the ground. This progression is known as the 'gait cycle.' Unyielding surfaces interrupt this normal gait cycle, again causing stress and micro-trauma to your plantar fascia.

Whether you are a professional athlete or someone wanting to take their first jog in 15 years, foot injuries as a result of exercise can be debilitating and cause you months of rehabilitation.

APC Injections Can Benefit All Not Just Professional Athletes

Published: 5-18-13

Like Tiger Woods and Kobe Bryant, Olympic long jump hopeful Norris Frederick recently turned to revolutionary Platelet-Rich Plasma (PRP) therapy to relieve his knee pain. The athlete reported significant relief after receiving PRP injections.

After suffering a knee injury, he was treated with a series of two injections of platelet-rich plasma over four weeks. The most significant initial subjective findings showed that he had reduced pain and moderate to significant increases in range of motion. Frederick plans to continue his quest for gold at the 2016 Olympic Games in Rio de Janeiro, Brazil.

A benefit of platelet-rich plasma therapy is that it heals and strengthens tendons and ligaments, strengthening and thickening the tissue up to 40 percent in some cases. This is different than the effects of Cortisone, which studies have shown may actually weaken tissue. Cortisone shots may provide temporary pain relief and stop inflammation, but they do not provide long-term healing.

I have used platelet-rich plasma injections for heel pain for many years in my practice. Platelet-rich plasma is blood plasma with concentrated platelets. The concentrated platelets contain huge reservoirs of bioactive proteins, including growth factors that are vital to initiate and accelerate tissue repair and regeneration. These bioactive proteins initiate connective tissue healing: bone, tendon and ligament regeneration and repair, promote development of new blood vessels, and stimulate wound healing.

My patients see a significant improvement in their symptoms and a remarkable return of function which may eliminate the need for more aggressive treatments such as long-term medication or surgery.

PRP injections can be performed in tendons and ligaments all over the body. Sports injuries, arthritic joints, lower back, degenerative disc disease and more specific injuries including tennis elbow, carpal tunnel syndrome, ACL tears, shin splints, rotator cuff tears, plantar fasciitis and iliotibial band syndrome may all be effectively treated with platelet-rich plasma.

Platelet-rich plasma therapy helps regenerate tendons and ligaments, but it is not a quick fix. This therapy is stimulating the growth and repair of tendons and ligaments and requires time and rehabilitation. Through regular visits, your doctor will determine when you are able to resume regular physical activities.

If you have a tendon or ligament injury and traditional methods have not provided relief, then platelet-rich plasma therapy may be the solution. The procedure is less aggressive and less expensive than surgery. It will heal tissue with minimal or no scarring and alleviates further degeneration of the tissues.

Talk to your doctor to see if platelet-rich plasma therapy is right for you.

Revolutionary Blood Platelet Injections

Published: 12-19-09

The most common foot condition that brings patients to my office is heel pain.

Heel pain is caused by the inflammation of the plantar fascia, multiple muscles, the bursa, nerves, and the periosteum under the heel.

For most people, heel pain is at its worst in the morning.

While you're sleeping, your feet rest in a downward, relaxed position, causing your muscles to tighten. When you take your first steps out of bed, stretching these tight muscles can cause pain.

You can also feel heel pain after prolonged standing and walking, which is why many people complain of sore heels after a long day on their feet.

In fact, most people feel more pain after standing than walking, because you have more tension on the plantar fascia while standing than during the actual movement of walking.

Last year alone, I saw almost 200 heel pain patients, and while I only performed heel surgery on about 1 percent of them, that was 1 percent too many!

Even though heel surgery is simple to perform, the recovery period can be long.

After heel surgery, the patient's foot is in a cast for four weeks before he or she will need extensive rehabilitation for two to four months.

Three years ago, I learned something that surprised many foot and ankle specialists: chronic inflammation can lead to the death of cells.

In light of this new discovery, I began injecting Autologous Platelet Concentrates into chronically inflamed areas with great success, as did many other doctors.

Your blood's platelets contain growth factors. This injection isolates the platelets from each patient's own blood and is then re-injected into the area of chronic inflammation.

With this therapy, recovery time is only two weeks. Plus, it has no side effects since it is the patient's own blood that we re-inject.

In addition, a local anesthetic is used on the injection site, so there is minimal pain. The entire procedure only takes about 15 minutes.

After this therapy, patients are required to wear a Cam Walker, also known as a walking boot, for two weeks. Healing continues over the next several weeks.

Also, the therapy can be repeated.

So far, this technique has been used for many kinds of chronic inflammation, such as chronically inflamed wounds, bones and tendons.

If you have any type of heel pain syndrome, an injection may be a great non-surgical approach to get you back to enjoying life's activities.

Heel Pain & Young Athletes

Published: *11-14-09*

Indoors and outdoors, young athletes stay active year-round in competitive sports. For many of them, heel pain has become another part of the game. When a child complains of heel pain, it should be diagnosed right away. It may be a warning sign of a serious foot problem. Heel pain often occurs in children ages 6-14 as their feet grow and the heel bone develops.

As children become more active in sports, they increase their risk for growth-plate injuries and subsequent heel pain. This is especially true at the beginning of the school year, when surgeons see an increase in middle school and high school athletes experiencing heel pain, since football and soccer are simultaneously underway. New bone forms in an area behind the heel, known as the growth plate, and cartilage is vulnerable to severe inflammation from strain or stress. With repeated stresses and strains from over-activity, the heel becomes painful.

Even though growth-plate trauma is the leading cause of heel pain in young people, the condition can be difficult to diagnose. Parents should be concerned if a child has pain in the back or bottom of the heel, limps, walks on the toes, or seems to have difficulty participating in normal recreational activities. The condition is diagnosed by a thorough examination of the child's feet and legs, and possible medical imaging tests to rule out other serious causes of heel pain, such as bursitis, tendonitis and fractures.

In most cases, mild or moderate heel pain can be treated with shoe inserts, anti-inflammatory medications, stretching, and physical therapy.

In severe cases, the foot and ankle will be immobilized in a cast. In some instances, surgery may be necessary. Heel pain in young people often returns after treatment since the growth plate is still forming until the age of 14 or 15. However, the risk for reoccurrence can be lowered by choosing well-constructed shoes with good support and restricting the use of spiked athletic shoes, especially on hard fields.

Young athletes should also avoid competition that exceeds their physical abilities. If your child is experiencing heel or foot pain, call a qualified podiatrist or foot specialist for an assessment.

Chapter 8

Gait Analysis and Correction

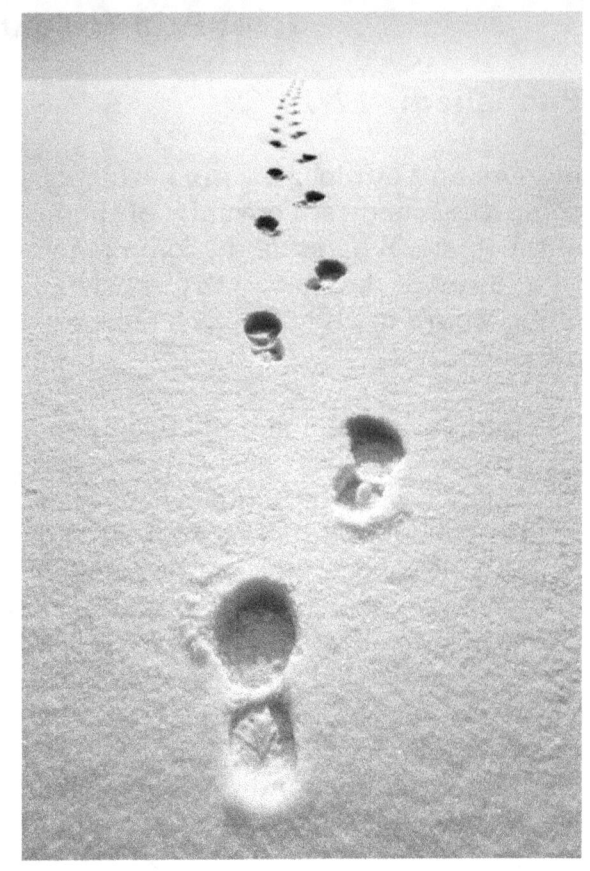

That Pain in Your Back Could be Linked to Your Feet!

Published: *3-23-13*

If your lower back has been hurting, and you don't remember doing anything to injure it, the source of your pain could be your feet.
Foot pain is something that many people try to ignore. After all, doesn't everyone's feet hurt now and then? But if foot pain is something that has been with you for quite awhile, it could be causing problems in your ankles, knees, hips and even your back.

That old song, "The leg bone's connected to the thigh bone...," tells the whole story. Our bodies are like a chain, with one link, or bone, connecting at the joint to another link.

Think about what would happen if the first link in the chain was out of position. The point at which it meets the next link would eventually overstress that link and adversely affect the entire chain.

That's what happens when we have foot pain. If the normal way of walking is painful, we instinctively change our walking pattern.
Say you have arthritis, and your big toe joint hurts. You change your gait to avoid bending the joint when you walk. Changing your gait changes the mechanics of your ankle joint, eventually causing ankle pain. This change in your walking pattern can also affect the whole chain of your lower body, from the ankle, to the knee, to the hip and then to the lower back.

When foot pain or a foot deformity causes you to change the way you walk, it changes the way the bones of all those other joints move with each other. Cartilage in the joints can wear down, ligaments and tendons can be stressed beyond their normal range and arthritis can set in.

A good way to check if your gait has changed is to check the wear pattern on your shoes. Here are some helpful hints:

- Even wear: If the treads on your shoes across the heel, and under the ball of the foot are both worn, with additional wear marks underneath the big toe, then this is a sign of a healthy stride.
- Edge wear: If your shoe has tread loss on the outside of the shoe and, in extreme instances, holes in the upper, this is a sign of a "supinator," or those who don't pronate or roll their ankles inward enough and strike the ground with the outside edges of their feet. High arches are a common cause of supination. This type of gait puts a lot of pressure on the leg and can cause stress fractures, especially in runners.
- Heel wear: Shoes that are worn in the heel down to the midsole show a person is overstriding when they walk. An overstride means that you walk with your feet too far in front of your body. Most of the rotation of the foot happens in the air and causes a lot of impact on the heel of the foot. Most walkers with this gait have plantar fasciitis or heel spur syndromes.
- Heel and forefoot wear: If there is significant wear in the heel extending to the ball of foot and big toe, then this is a sign of overpronation. People with flat arches and very flexible feet have this wear pattern. Custom orthotics are a very good option for this type of foot problem.

If your feet or ankles aren't working right, your shoes will probably be a great clue. Don't ignore them! Contact a foot and ankle specialist for an evaluation. Caught early, most foot pain and deformities can be treated conservatively. Your back (and knees and hips) will thank you!

Flat Feet: Causes, Surgical Treatments and Beneficial Exercises- Question and Answer

Published: *12-1-12*

Q: Can you discuss flat feet?

A: Fallen arches, or flat feet, are a legitimate medical condition affecting about 5 percent of Americans. Flat feet can be present at birth or develop over decades of walking, running and overall time spent on the feet, especially on hard surfaces in the workplace.

There are several types of flatfoot conditions that occur in adults.

The most common type is adult-acquired flatfoot. It is caused by overstretching a tendon that supports the arch.

Another common type is flexible flatfoot, in which the foot is flat when standing, but returns to a normal arch in non-weight-bearing positions.

Flat feet can be very painful and make people avoid walking, running and exercise. But if you seek medical attention early, a foot and ankle surgeon may be able to prevent it from becoming a more serious foot problem.

A flat foot can actually be a tendon tear, fracture, or another disorder, like Charcot neuroarthropathy, so a complete podiatric exam, including x-rays, should be done to evaluate your condition.

Treatments may include modifying or limiting activities, stretching exercises, custom shoe inserts and non-steroidal anti-inflammatory medications.

If those techniques don't work, a variety of surgical procedures may be considered to relieve pain and improve foot function.

Q: Are drugstore-quality arch supports worthwhile?

A: To be truly effective, an orthotic must be fitted for your particular needs. This means that a casting or 3-D digital scan of your foot must be completed to get a true picture of your foot.

Scanners at your big-box retailer only take a "pressure point" picture of your foot, not a 3-D image. A 3-D image or casting is sent to a laboratory where a custom orthotic device is fabricated to the exact specifications of your podiatrist.

Your podiatrist will take into account your particular foot problems in writing the prescription for the laboratory. A functional orthotic controls foot movement and helps a person walk in a way that best supports joints and muscles.

Wearing an ill-fitted orthotic is not only a waste of time, but it can also make your foot problems worse. Over time, these problems can lead to leg, knee, hip, and even back problems. Store-bought orthotics tend to offer relief and comfort for only a short period of time.

Q: Other than flip flops and thongs, are there other types of shoes to avoid?

A: Any shoe that can be bent in the middle is not a good choice for someone with flat feet. This includes ballet type shoes, dock shoes and high heel pumps.

The key factors to remember are that the shoe should have stability, support and motion control. When looking at shoe reviews or technical specifications, any indication of "added support" means you are headed in the right direction.

The main technology found in stability shoes is a medial post of dual density foam. Footwear producers inject a harder compound of foam right below the medial side of the arch and sometimes extended all the way to the heel. It is easily recognizable as a darker, almost always gray, piece of foam on the inside of the midsole.

Q: What exercises can be of value?

A: Three exercises that can be of value in keeping the arch healthy are the towel scrunch, stair raise for arch strength and the can roll.

With time and decreased demand, the small muscles of your arch become weaker. The muscles lose their ability to give your feet the spring they once had.

To strengthen those muscles, start with the "towel scrunch" by placing a small hand towel on the floor and reaching out with your toes to grab the towel and scrunch it back toward you, bunching it up under your foot. Keep reaching out and grabbing more towel until you run out.

At the end of each scrunch, hold the contraction you feel in the arch for just a second before releasing. I recommend three sets daily.

The toe raise can be done on a stair or raised board at least four inches from the ground. Stand on the stair with only the ball of your foot and rise up to your tiptoes, pressing down with your toes. When you lower, resist the urge to drop your heel too far below the stair or raised board. This becomes a calf exercise, and you want to focus on your arch. Do 10 of these per set and three sets a day.

Finish you arch routine with a good flexibility exercise. Sitting in your favorite chair, place the arch of your foot on a soup can, turned on its side, and, with your foot, roll it freely away and back from you from the ball of your foot to your heel. This stretches and massages the bottom of the foot and can be a way to reduce some arch soreness.

Q: What are some criteria used to determine if surgery is needed?

A: If you have had prolonged pain that is not helped with conservative methods, and your abnormal gait causes pain in other parts of your body such as your knees and back, then surgery may be your only option.

Surgery for flat feet is invasive and requires a long recuperation period, sometimes up to one year. Each individual case will be evaluated and may involve several procedures including one or more of the following: posterior tibia tendon repair, F.D.L. tendon transfer, calcaneal osteotomy, lateral column lengthening, iliac aspiration and gastroc release.

Q: At what age would surgery be appropriate?

A: It can be difficult to tell if a child has flat feet as the arches don't fully develop until the age of 10. Before age 3, all children have flat feet.

The arch of the foot does not start to develop until about 3 years of age.

Older children may have flat feet for a number of reasons. Problems with ligaments, muscles, joints, bones, and the nervous system are all possible causes. Children with conditions such as Down, Marfan or Ehlers-Danlos syndromes are more likely to have flat feet.

Flatfoot Disorders and Current Treatment

Published: *8-20-11*

Treatment and prevention of adult flatfoot can reduce the incidence of additional foot problems such as bunions, hammertoes, arthritis and calluses. And, it can improve a person's overall health.

To tell if you have flat feet, wet your feet and stand on a flat, dry surface that will leave an imprint of your foot. A normal footprint has a wide band connecting the ball of the foot to the heel, with an indentation on the inner side of the foot. A foot with a high arch has a large indentation and a very narrow connecting band.

Flat feet leave a nearly complete imprint with almost no inward curve where the arch should be. Although you can do the "wet test" at home, a thorough examination by a doctor will be needed to identify why the flatfoot developed. Causes include a congenital abnormality, a bone fracture or dislocation, a torn or stretched tendon, arthritis or neurologic weakness.

An inability to rise up on your toes while standing on the affected foot may indicate damage to the posterior tibial tendon, which supports the heel and forms the arch. If "too many toes" show on the outside of your foot when the doctor views you from the rear, your shinbone (tibia) may be sliding off the anklebone (talus), another indicator of damage to the posterior tibial tendon. Be sure to wear your regular shoes to the examination. An irregular wear pattern on the bottom of the shoe is another indicator of acquired adult flatfoot. Your physician may request X-rays to see how the bones of your feet are aligned. Muscle and tendon strength are tested by asking you to move the foot while the doctor holds it.

Overweight males in white-collar jobs are most apt to suffer from adult flatfoot disorder, a progressive condition characterized by partial or total collapse of the arch, according to research. Symptoms of adult flatfoot include pain, swelling, flattening of the arch and an inward rolling of the ankle. Because flatfoot is a progressive disorder by nature, neglecting treatment or preventive care can lead to arthritis, loss of function of the foot and other painful foot disorders. In many cases, flatfoot can be treated with non-surgical approaches. A painless flatfoot that does not hinder your ability to walk or wear shoes requires no special treatment. Other treatment options depend on the cause and progression of the flatfoot.

Conservative treatment options include:

- Making shoe modifications.
- Using orthotic devices, such as arch supports and custom made orthoses.
- Taking non-steroidal anti-inflammatory drugs, such as ibuprofen, to relieve pain.
- Using a short-leg walking cast or wearing a brace.
- Injecting a corticosteroid into the joint to relieve pain.
- Rest and ice.
- Physical therapy.

Flatfoot disorder may gradually worsen to the point that many of the tendons and ligaments in the foot and ankle are simply overworking, often to the point where they tear and/or rupture. In some patients whose pain is not adequately relieved by conservative treatments, there are surgical techniques available to correct flatfoot and improve foot function, which can help reduce pain and improve bone alignment.

As in most progressive foot disorders, early treatment for flatfoot disorder is also the patient's best route for optimal success in controlling symptoms and additional damage to the feet. The goal is to keep patients active, healthy and as pain free as possible.

Read Your Footprints and How You Roll

Published: 7-3-10

Read your footprints and discover how you roll! Like a good detective story, your bare footprints can leave clues to your foot health and drop hints about possible problems. Before we crack the barefoot code, here's a quick course on walking patterns.

- The heel usually hits the ground first.
- As the foot moves forward, the arch flattens and weight is transferred to the ball of the foot.
- As you push off from the ball of the foot, the arch springs upward and does not touch the ground.

At least that's how normal feet are supposed to work. Unfortunately, many feet aren't normal. In normal feet, this movement is straight. If the foot rolls to the inside, it's called "overpronation" and can strain the arch and hurt the knee. If the foot rolls to the outside, it's called "underpronation" and can lead to stress fractures and ankle sprains.

Now, wet your bare feet, take a walk, and look at your footprints. If you see a large, oblong wet mark with toe prints and little or no dry, curved-in arch area, then you're overpronating or have flat feet. If there's little connection between the heel and front part of the foot, like a big dry area in the middle, it's likely you are underpronating or have a high arch. This means a lot of your weight is landing on the outside edge of your foot.

Athletic shoes with stability features are built with extra cushioning to remedy this problem. If you are prone to ankle sprains, wear high-top athletic shoes that cover the foot and ankle snugly to minimize damage from twists. Custom-molded arch supports will correct your abnormal or irregular walking pattern. In fact, the use of foot orthotics is quite common and is often compared to using eyeglasses. Just as eyeglasses correct your vision, orthotics bring your feet back into the correct position and help the alignment of your body. Custom-molded orthotics are made from a cast of the foot or new 3-D imaging of the foot. With 3-D digital scanning of your foot, podiatrists are able to get a more accurate custom orthotic without all the mess of plaster casting.

Do not be deceived by the "custom fit" orthotic stations in retail stores. Their scans only show how your weight is distributed based on a pressure scan. Then, an off-the-shelf, pre-fabricated orthotic is either suggested or mailed to you. True 3-D imaging of your foot creates a multi-dimensional digital image, which is used to fabricate a custom orthotic that is specific to your individual needs, including marking trouble spots for padding, pockets and other accommodations.

Anyone can make use of foot orthotics, even those who have no major foot problems. This is because orthotics can also be used to improve foot performance, which can be useful for people who stand and move a lot like dancers and athletes. Once you see how you "roll," talk with your podiatrist about custom-molded arch supports and footwear choices to reduce the potential damage from a rolling gait.

Chapter 9

Men's Foot Health

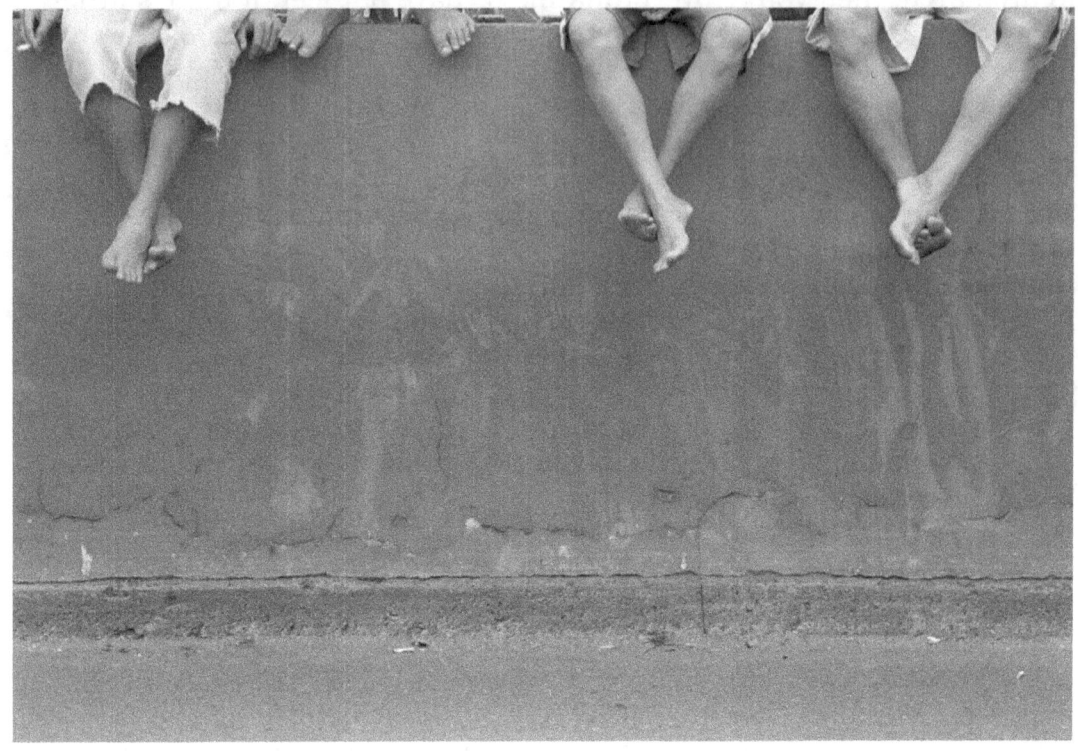

Top 10 Men's Foot Problems and Treatments

Published: *2-9-13*

Feet are the Rodney Dangerfield of body parts: "They don't get no respect!" That's especially true for men's feet. Men's feet and ankles take a beating with jobs that often require long hours standing or walking on hard surfaces such as concrete. Men often resist going to the doctor when they're sick or in pain until it starts slowing them down.

This Valentine's day, think of your husband's feet. Despite what many men tell themselves, foot pain is not normal. Here are my top 10 men's foot problems:

1. Heel pain is often caused by tissue inflammation, but can also result from a broken bone, a tight achilles tendon, a pinched nerve or other problem. A qualified physician will know how to diagnose

and treat the true cause of heel pain. Usually, heel pain is plantar fasciitis and this is successfully treated with conservative treatments by your physician.
2. Ankle sprains always, always, always require a prompt visit to the doctor. Participating in sports activities is one way men can get a sprained ankle, but even day-to-day activities such as walking on an uneven surface or slipping on an icy sidewalk can produce the painful stretching or tearing of the ankle ligament.
3. Hallux Rigidus, or big toe stiffness and pain, develops slowly over time as cartilage in the big toe joint wears down. This eventually leads to arthritis. The sooner a man has this diagnosed, the easier it is to treat. Golfers may develop it as a result of the motion of the foot during the follow-through of the swing, and other men may have jobs that increase the stress on the big toe, such as those requiring frequent stooping or squatting.
4. Achilles tendonitis usually develops from a sudden increase in physical activity, such as when unconditioned men play weekend sports. Chances of an achilles tendon rupture can be reduced by treatment of the symptoms of achilles tendonitis: pain and tenderness on the back of the foot or heel. These problems are also common in men whose work puts stress on their ankles and feet, such as laborers.
5. Ingrown toenails can pierce the skin, open the door for bacteria to enter the body, and convince some men to perform dangerous "bathroom surgery." Few men know that a doctor can perform a quick procedure that will end the pain and permanently cure an ingrown toenail.
6. Toe and metatarsal fractures (broken toes). Some people say that "the doctor can't do anything for a broken bone in the foot." This is usually not true. In fact, if a fractured toe or metatarsal bone is not treated correctly, serious complications may develop.
7. Athlete's foot is a chronic infection caused by various types of fungus. Athlete's foot is often spread in places where men go barefoot such as public showers or swimming pools. The condition ranges from mild scaling and itching to painful inflammation and blisters. It usually starts between the toes or on the arch and may spread to the bottom and sides of the foot. Depending on the type of infection, various kinds of medication may be used in treating a fungal problem. Successful treatment usually involves a combination of medication and self-care. If your condition is not serious, over-the-counter and prescription powders, lotions, or ointments can often help treat scaling, itching, and inflammation. Foot soaks may help dry excessive perspiration, especially ones with tea tree oil. If his athlete's foot does not improve, he may need to be prescribed stronger medication by a doctor.

8. Onychomycosis, or fungal nails, refers to any number of fungal infections that can occur on the nails of the feet. I see a lot of men with this condition due to sweaty feet, poor hygiene and tight fitting shoes. Fungus that occurs on nails is usually more resistant and more difficult to treat than athlete's foot, so physician formula topical or oral antifungal medications may be prescribed. Few men know that laser therapy is available now for fungal nails and is a great option since oral medications have risky side-effects.
9. Foot warts are harmless, even though they may be painful. Men often mistake warts for corns or calluses, which are layers of dead skin that build up to protect an area which is being continuously irritated. A wart, however, is caused by a viral infection which invades the skin through small or invisible cuts and abrasions. Foot warts are generally raised and fleshy and can appear anywhere on the feet or toes. Occasionally, warts can spontaneously disappear after a short time, and then, just as frequently, they recur in the same location. If left untreated, warts can grow to an inch or more in circumference and can spread into clusters of warts. A raised bump on his foot should always be evaluated by a podiatrist as warts are very contagious.
10. Men's footwear has come a long way since Roman armies conquered an empire wearing only sandals on their feet! But what's old is new again as more and more men wear sandals...even in the winter! Along with the growing popularity of men's sandals come more aches and pains for male feet. The wrong sandal could cause problems including stress fractures in some of the foot's 26 bones. I recommend men wear a man sandal-or the 'mandal' as some people call it! Look for a sturdy, cushioned, supportive sole and padded straps. Men with diabetes should consult their foot and ankle surgeon before wearing any type of sandal.

If the man in your life has any of these symptoms, let him know it is not normal and he should see a podiatrist. If caught early most of the above conditions can be treated very successfully. After all he should know...happy wife, happy life!

Chapter 10

Skin Conditions of the Feet

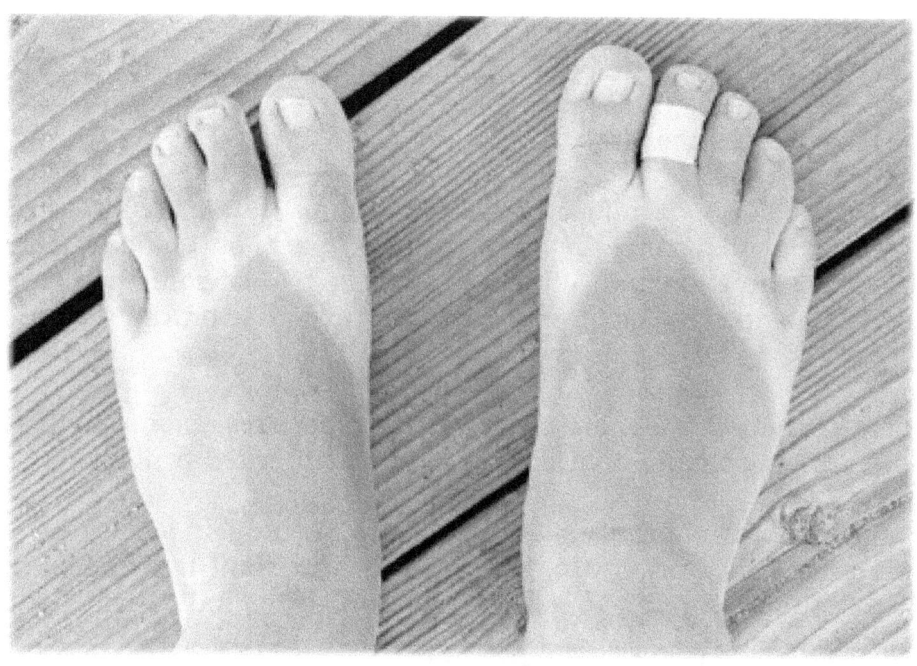

Diagnosis of Melanoma Saves Lives

Published: *11-10-12*

Recently, in Forbes Life magazine, an article on Debra Black, wife of private equity billionaire Leon Black, and her fight against melanoma was documented.

Mrs. Black noticed a growth on the bottom of her foot and quickly showed it to her dermatologist. Debra had the earliest form of skin cancer seven years before, so she diligently went for screenings every few months.

Her doctor, one of New York City's top-rated dermatologists, told her not to worry and that it was just a plantar wart. He froze it off. It came back. He cut it off. It came back. It hurt and eventually bled. For four years, her doctor insisted it was nothing.

Black wasn't convinced. In early 2007, she went to a friend's podiatrist, who ordered a 3-D sonogram.

It turned out that she had stage II melanoma. Had she waited much longer, she might have died.

After two skin grafts, six weeks of keeping her foot elevated above her pelvis for 23 hours a day, and four months of using a walker and wheelchair, she was cancer-free.

We often view the sun's harmful rays as the primary cause of skin cancer due to the fact that this cancer is often found on parts of the body that receive the most sun exposure. While this may be true of some bodily skin cancers, this does not hold true for those that arise on the skin of the feet.

Skin cancers of the feet are more often related to viruses, exposure to chemicals, chronic inflammation or irritation, or inherited traits.

Unfortunately, the skin of the feet is often overlooked during routine medical examinations, and for this reason, it is important that the feet are checked regularly for abnormalities which might be indicative of evolving skin cancer.

Skin cancers of the feet have several features in common. Most are painless and often there is a history of recurrent cracking, bleeding or ulceration. Frequently, individuals discover their skin cancer after unrelated ailments near the affected site. Some of the most common cancers of the lower extremity are basal, squamous and malignant melanoma.

Hear are the ABCDs of melanoma's attributes of cancerous lesions:

- **A**symmetry: If divided in half, the sides don't match.

- **B**orders: They look scalloped, uneven or ragged.

- **C**olor: They may have more than one color. These colors may have an uneven distribution.

- **D**iameter: They can appear wider than a pencil eraser, greater than 6 millimeters.

For other types of skin cancer, look for spontaneous ulcers and non-healing sores, bumps that crack or bleed, nodules with rolled or "donut-shaped" edges, or a discrete scaly area. If you notice a mole, bump or patch on your skin or the skin of a friend or family member that meets any of these criteria, encourage them to see a podiatrist. Your podiatrist will investigate the possibility of skin cancer both through his/her clinical examination and with the use of a skin biopsy.

A skin biopsy is a simple procedure in which a small sample of the skin lesion is obtained and sent to a specialized laboratory where a skin pathologist will examine the tissue in greater detail.

To ensure that you receive the very best in care, your podiatrist will likely require that your skin biopsy be sent to a lab with board-certified dermatopathologists who have specialized training in the analysis of abnormal skin lesions from the lower leg and foot.

If a lesion is determined to be malignant, your podiatrist will recommend the best course of treatment for your condition. It could save your life.

Flesh Eating Bacteria and Tips to Save Your Feet

Published: 7-7-12

If you have been paying attention to the news, you have probably heard the name Aimee Copeland. If the name doesn't sound familiar, have you heard about flesh-eating bacteria in the news recently? Aimee, 24, has been fighting flesh-eating bacteria for several weeks.

At the beginning of May, the University of West Georgia graduate student fell from a homemade zip line. She ended up with a gash in her left calf. The gash was treated and closed with 22 staples, but, within days, Aimee developed a serious infection. The infection was so serious that doctors had to amputate both of Aimee's hands, a leg and remove tissue from her torso. Aimee was also put on a ventilator and she experienced organ failure.

The media says that Aimee has flesh-eating bacteria. The correct medical term for Aimee's condition is necrotizing fasciitis. Necrotizing fasciitis is a rare, but very serious condition. It occurs when bacteria gets into the tissue that surround muscles, nerves and blood vessels. Once in the body, the bacteria produce toxins that shut down the immune system. With the body's defense system out of service, the bacteria can destroy skin, fat and muscle very quickly. It is like the bacteria are eating away at the body. This is why it is called "flesh-eating bacteria." The bacteria can also get into the blood and spread to the organs, causing failure.

Many types of bacteria can cause necrotizing fasciitis. Two common bacteria that cause the disease are Streptococcus pyogenes (Group A strep) and Staphylococcus aureus.

Aimee's necrotizing fasciitis was caused by Aeromonas hydrophilia. This bacterium is found in almost all freshwater sources and is not usually dangerous to humans. However, Aeromonas hydrophilia is hard to treat with antibiotics, and if it gets into the tissue, it can be very damaging. Knowing that there is flesh-eating bacteria out there is very scary. Necrotizing fasciitis can happen to anyone, even healthy people. Some people do have a higher risk such as diabetics, people with open sores or people who have weakened immune systems due to age, cancer or chemotherapy. The best thing you can do to protect yourself from necrotizing fasciitis is to seek quick medical attention.

Do not hesitate to make an appointment with your podiatrist or any medical facility for proper treatment of cuts, wounds, sores, gashes and/or burns on your feet. The next thing you should do is pay attention to your feet. If the pain is getting worse, don't hesitate to contact your podiatrist again or go to the emergency room.

Necrotizing fasciitis develops very quickly. If the disease spreads too fast, doctors will have to amputate parts of the body to stop the infection from reaching vital organs. The sooner doctors are able to diagnose you and start treatment, the better your chances of keeping all of your toes.

Aimee's story is horrible, but there is good news. Aimee appears to be making progress. As we all hope for Aimee's recovery, let's also learn from her story. With the summer ahead, our bare feet will be exposed to all kinds of things, including bacteria. Remember to be safe, practice proper foot care, and see your podiatrist immediately if any injuries should occur. Acting quickly can save a limb and your life.

Chapter 11

Shoes and the Proper Fit

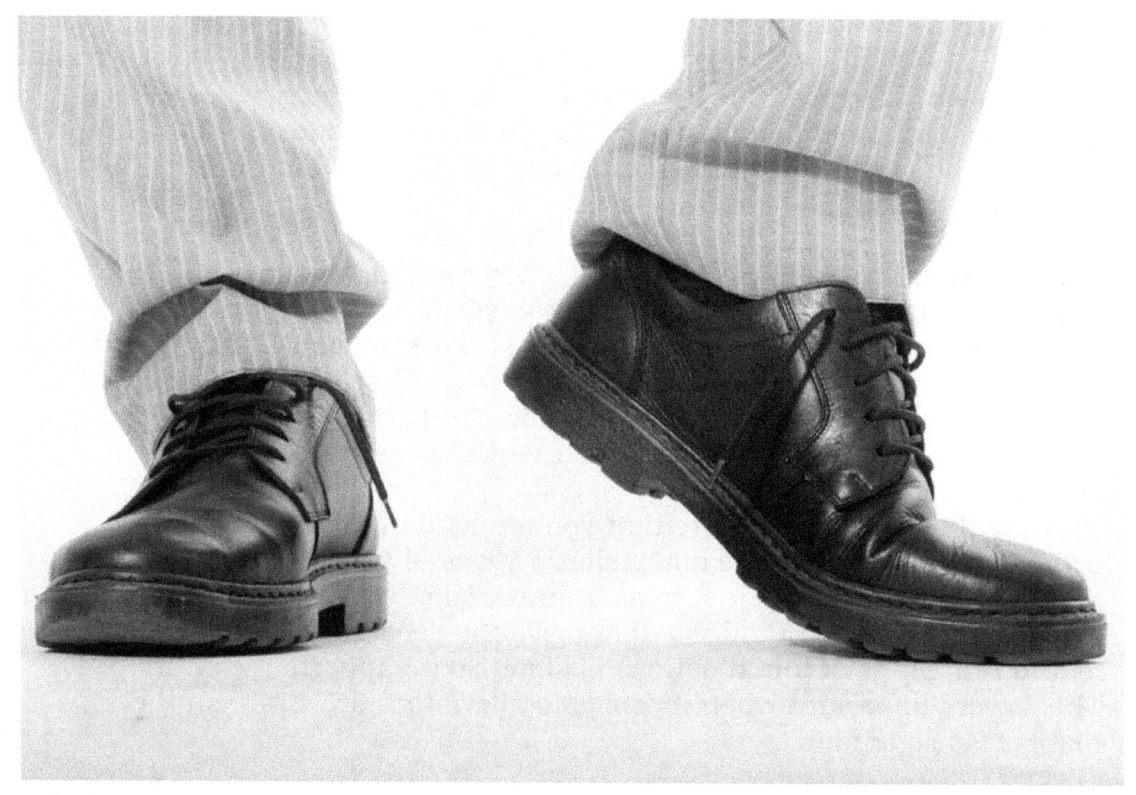

Flip Flop Injuries in Young Adults

Published: *6-16-12*

After months wearing boots and thick-soled shoes, many are welcoming the warmer weather sporting flip-flop sandals. However, their popularity among teens and young adults is responsible for a growing epidemic of heel pain and foot deformities.

We are seeing more heel pain than ever in patients 15 to 25 years old, a group that usually doesn't have this problem. A major contributor is wearing flip-flops with paper-thin soles every day throughout the summer.

Flip-flops have no arch support and can accentuate any abnormal biomechanics in foot motion, and this eventually brings pain and inflammation. Flip-flops also cause tension in the foot from the motion of lifting the heel away from the shoe surface, that flip-flop sound that you can't miss.

This tension, along with no arch support, brings on the type of heel pain caused by chronic inflammation of the connective tissue extending from the heel bone to the toes, the plantar fascia. This heel pain is also known as plantar fasciitis.

Plantar fasciitis pain is most noticeable after getting out of bed in the morning, and it tends to decrease after a few minutes and returns during the day as time on the feet increases. Most patients with plantar fasciitis respond to conservative treatment within six weeks. This can consist of stretching exercises, night splints, padding and strapping of the foot, custom orthotics and anti-inflammatory medicines.

You should always make sure that you are actually getting a custom orthotic made from a three dimensional image of your foot, not the over-the-counter brands that just take an impression of the bottom of your foot. These types of orthotics will not give the necessary correction in the foot to bring it back into a neutral position so it supports the entire body. This is very important when it comes to alleviating the strain on the plantar fascia tendon.

I also see many patients with ankle sprains from the strain of wearing a non-supportive shoe like flip-flops.

Increased overuse injuries to the feet, and ankles in particular, can lead to more problems in the rest of your body including the knee, hip and back. If the foundation of your body, your feet, is not supported and in alignment, then the rest of your body will not be either.

Another common ailment in patients who wear flip-flops everyday is hammertoes.

The disfiguring condition is caused by the scrunching motion of your toes when you walk and leads to strain and deformity of the bones in the toes.

Beware of wearing flip-flops while driving. They can become lodged under the gas pedal or brake or slip off while you're driving. Also, make sure you do not wear flip-flops while riding a bike. I had a patient loose a toe from colliding into a car while wearing flip-flops.

I advise wearing sandals with reasonably strong soles and arch support. Thicker-soled sandals with supportive arches might not be considered stylish for girls and young women. But if you want to wear sandals most of the time, you'll avoid heel pain and other foot deformities if you choose sturdier, perhaps less-fashionable, styles.

Rock & Roll for Your Feet: Will Toning Shoes Give You That Rockin' Body?

Published: *3-5-11*

Tone your legs! Strengthen your core! Improve your posture! Get a better body without putting in any extra effort! That sounds good. Or maybe too good to be true. These are some of the claims made by athletic shoe companies now producing toning shoes.

But before you put down the big bucks for the newest fad in shoes, you may want more information.

First, let me give you an overview of rocker shoes. There are actually several different types of shoes that may employ some instability or a rocking motion to varying degrees.

Toning shoes may look odd but claim to utilize various designs to force the core muscles in your body to work harder to obtain balance. They usually have significant 1-inch or more rounded soles and extra cushioning to alter the wearer's normal walking gait.

Also called unstable rocker shoes, these shoes are designed to induce instability in all planes of motion.

The idea is that if you walk in an unstable shoe, your body is forced to adapt, thus simulating the effect of walking on soft, uneven terrain. Your core muscles are strengthened as your body adapts to the instability of the shoe.

Masai Barefoot Technology pioneered this concept, but brands like Skechers, Reebok, Joya and Z7 now have toning shoes.

Mild rocker shoes are not meant to change posture or balance. They reduce strain on the heel and toes by allowing you to roll normally with each step. You see this design in most diabetic shoe manufacturers such as Dr. Comfort, Natural Step and Aetrex.

Stable and medical rockers are great for reducing certain motion in the toe joints or taking pressure away from a particular area of the foot. These are mainly prescribed by podiatrists to treat arthritis or pain in the ball of the foot, diabetes and plantar fasciitis. People who over-pronate or have unstable feet tend to feel much better in a stable rocker-sole shoe. They also may be prescribed for use after surgical procedures.

I encourage the use of custom or over-the-counter orthotics in stable rocker-sole shoes to achieve the greatest amount of stability and control. Brands like RYN, Finn Comfort "Finnamic," Mephisto Sano and Cogent are all good examples of stable rocker shoes.

Recently, commercials for toning shoes claim you can "burn more calories, tone muscles, improve posture and reduce joint stress wearing these shoes." They also claim "the shoe is proven to work your hamstrings and calves up to 11 percent harder and tones your butt up to 28 percent more than regular sneakers just by walking."

In light of these lofty claims, the University of Wisconsin-La Crosse enlisted a team of exercise scientists to study these shoes.

The results across the board showed no statistically significant increases in either exercise response or muscle activation during any of the treadmill tests. There is simply no evidence to support the claims that these shoes will burn more calories and improve muscle strength and tone.

Also, toning shoes can change your walking or standing posture. They can change how you walk and the muscles of the body adjust and compensate. Because you will be using different muscles when you first wear these shoes, you're probably going to be sore. But remember, if you wear any shoe that is abnormally shaped that you are not use to wearing, it is naturally going to make your muscles sore. This is not going to translate into toning your hamstrings and butt.

In some people, toning shoes can cause injuries such as achilles tendinitis or ankle sprains because they change your standing posture. But in others, the slight adjustment in gait can feel good. This can be deceptive though, because you are walking on an inch worth of cushioning in these shoes.

It is important also to remember that anyone who already has an unstable gait or previous knee, hip or back problems should be very cautious about using toning shoes. Because your standing posture is altered with this type of shoe, it can put extra pressure on these areas of your body and cause more harm than good.

Most doctors agree that if these shoes can get people motivated to walk, thereby improving their health and fitness, they can be worth the money.

However, make sure to check with your podiatrist who can recommend the best shoe for any activity. Also, be sure to wear them in gradually and stop immediately if any pain or discomfort develops.

Always remember there is nothing that takes the place of a good exercise regime that utilizes both cardiovascular and strength training. With this information at hand, and if you still want to give the toning shoe fad a try, the American Podiatric Medical Association has granted their seal of acceptance to the Reebok Easytone due to its less rounded sole, which offers more stability than the other manufacturers.

High Heeled Shoe Damage and Simple Tips for Prevention

Published: 1-22-11

Women have been wearing high-heeled shoes since the 1800s, when shoes were made to match the outfit. Today, women wear high heels to make their legs look longer and their ankles thinner and, yes, sexy.

As a podiatrist, I see women every day complaining of pain in their feet. Often, they attribute their pain to an exercise regimen or their athletic shoes. After a thorough exam of their feet, I often find the shoes they are using for athletic activities are not the problem. It's the shoes they wear to work every day!

It's unrealistic for me to expect women not to wear fashionable, trendy shoes, but you may want to think twice about wearing them every day. You could be causing more damage to your feet than you know.

Wearing high heels changes the biomechanics of walking, and can have an impact on the entire structure of the foot and the relationship of the knee to the ankle, as well as your lower back. It puts more pressure on your feet per square inch. This means if you are overweight and wearing high heels, you will put a lot of added pressure per square inch on your feet as you walk.

High-heeled shoes have been linked to many foot ailments like bunions, hammertoes, neuromas, metatarsalgia, Achilles tendonitis, ingrown toenails, corns and calluses. It also affects the veins in your legs by effecting the blood circulation.

If you wear a heel that is more than 1½ inches high every day, your calf muscle will not effectively pump blood out of the leg. You can try this at home. Feel how the calf contracts when you walk in lower heels and then switch to high heels. The foot simply moves forward in high heels without your calf contracting. This can lead to the development of varicose veins.

So, what is a fashion-conscious woman to do? Try these simple steps to minimize the damage to your feet from high-heeled shoes:

- **Get your shoes fitted to your feet properly.** Most women wear shoes that are a half-size too small. Measure your feet with a brannock device every time you go shoe shopping to make sure your shoe size hasn't changed. Even a few extra pounds will cause your foot size to increase. Remember that different shoe manufacturers will size differently. Don't be a slave to your shoe-size number. Always make sure the shoe is the correct width. The shoes will not stretch that much when you "break it in." Most of my patients buy shoes that are too narrow.

- **Buy shoes in the afternoon or at the end of the day.** Your feet swell throughout the day, so you will get a better, more realistic fit if you buy in the afternoon.

- **Buy leather shoes, not synthetics.** Leather is a natural material that conforms to your foot more easily than synthetic materials.

- **Wear heels that are no higher than three inches and beware of the pointy-toed, high-heeled stiletto shoe.** These are a double-whammy. Try to avoid the severe point and go for more of a taper or square-toe box and a chunkier heel. I've seen women who surgically alter their feet to accommodate the severe taper of high heeled shoes.

- **Also, try to wear a consistent heel height as variations can cause pain in your Achilles tendon.** Chronic wear of high-heeled shoes causes a shortening of the Achilles tendon. This shortening can lead to tendonitis and heel pain. To combat this, stretch your Achilles tendon and calf muscles at least every day if not twice a day.

- **Wear your heels less than three hours a day.** Giving your feet a rest from the constriction of high heeled shoes is important. If your feet are swollen and painful after wearing your heels, that's an indication you're wearing them too long. This can cause severe problems including bunions and hammering of the toes. Bunions are bony growths at the base of the big toe. Your large toe separates from your foot and can cause excruciating pain when it gets into advanced stages. The big toe will angle inward toward the other toes and the bump can become swollen, inflamed, painful and unsightly.

Hammertoes will develop because the shoes will force the toes to crumple up. This shortens the muscles inside and leaves them permanently bent.

You may also experience the "pump bump." This is where the straps and the rigid backs of pump style shoes cause a bony enlargement on the heel.

It can also cause plantar (ball of foot) fasciitis, which, over time as it develops can become extremely painful and require treatment by your podiatrist including surgery.

If you have bunions or hammertoes, a silicone protective sleeve can help alleviate the pain and rubbing in your shoes. Hammertoes and bunions have to be corrected surgically to stop the pain it causes when you wear shoes, especially heels.

- If you have constant knee pain, avoid heels all together. One study showed a 26 percent increase in stress on the knee joint in heels higher than two inches. Osteoarthritis in the knee has been linked to chronic wearing of high heel shoes.

- If you have two different-sized feet, and most people do, shoe stretchers can be used to stretch the toe box if one foot is only a little bigger than the other. Remember though, you can only stretch 100-percent leather. If you have significantly different sized feet, some stores and web sites will sell you two different sized shoes.

- If you have to wear heels and have a flexible flat foot, try custom orthotics made especially for dress shoes. They can distribute weight off the ball of the foot back to the heel. This weight shift improves body alignment and balance dramatically, reducing leg and lower back fatigue while reducing pressure on the ball of the foot. It also helps relieve forefoot pressure from painful metatarsal heads, Morton's neuroma and calluses.

- Always have a pair of comfortable casual or athletic shoes handy at your desk or in the trunk of your car. Change into these shoes if you are sitting at work for long periods of time.

- Core strengthening exercises can help stabilize your feet and decrease the stress from high heeled shoes. Every woman should do core exercises at least three times a week. They help with back pain, knee pain and foot pain caused by instability.

It's important to realize that your feet were never designed to wear high heels. Think before you wear the latest trend-setting style. A few aches and pains are normal with high-heeled shoes. If you have pain that lasts more than five days see your podiatrist. It could indicate you're damaging your feet.

If caught early, simple solutions are available at your podiatrist's office, but if you delay treatment then more expensive surgical treatments may be needed to correct the damage to your feet.

Back to School Shoe Tips

Published: *8-7-10*

Kids are heading back to school soon and, of course, everyone wants new shoes. While flip-flops are all the rage for the beach and the pool, they can create problems in crowded school hallways and getting on and off the school bus.

While it may not be easy to coax your kids out of flip-flops for school, it's safer for them to wear a shoe with more support. Don't let fashion take a front seat to practicality and safety.

Your podiatrist can recommend some great options for teenagers that may fit the bill in the fashion area while still providing support and comfort throughout the day. To help busy parents with shoe choices, I recommend some simple guidelines to prevent or minimize possible foot problems from inappropriate shoes, such as painful ingrown toenails, blisters, heel pain and flat feet.

Kids come in all shapes and sizes, and so do their shoes. Shop at stores with experienced sales people that feature a wide selection of footwear styles, sizes and widths. Do not assume a given size will fit the same for different brands of shoes.

When choosing kids' shoes, size and shock absorption are the key considerations, especially if your child has flat feet that can worsen from improper fitting or worn-out shoes. Also, a child's foot can grow a size or two within a few months, so it's critical to allow room for growth in the toe box, about a finger's width from the longest toe.

If your children will be participating in sports this Fall, send them onto the field or the court with properly fitted shoes that are designed for the specific sport they are playing. Basketball shoes, for example, are designed for quick stops and starts, and ankle support, while a football cleat needs to serve an entirely different purpose. Let the shoe fit the sport and try to get help when choosing shoes for each sport.

Avoid man-made materials, like rubber and plastic, because they limit breathability. Hand-me-down clothes are great, but not shoes.

Once you've purchased those new shoes, remember to check them every several months, since kids' feet grow rapidly. Snug shoes can put pressure on the toes, causing ingrown nails, which is when a nail compresses and grows down into the skin. Infection can occur when an ingrown nail breaks through the skin. If there's pain, redness and fluid draining from the area, it's probably infected.

The ingrown nail can be removed in a simple, in-office procedure. Don't try to remove a child's ingrown nail at home. This can cause the condition to worsen. Tight-fitting shoes also cause blisters, corns and calluses on the toes and blisters on the back of the heels.

Never buy shoes that feel tight and uncomfortable in the store. Don't assume they will stretch or break in over time. Conversely, shoes that are too loose can cause problems, too. If a shoe is too loose, the foot can slide forward and put excessive pressure on the toes.

I recommend parents carefully inspect both new and old shoes to check for proper cushioning and arch support. Shoes lose their shock absorption over time, and wear and tear around the edges of the sole usually indicates it's worn out and should be replaced.

If a child keeps wearing worn-out or non-supportive dress or athletic shoes, it elevates the risk for developing heel pain, Achilles tendonitis and even ankle sprains and stress fractures. A good tip for parents when buying new shoes: The toe box should flex easily and the shoe shouldn't bend in the middle of the sole.

For children with flat feet, parents should buy oxford, lace-up shoes that have enough depth for an orthotic insert, if necessary. Unfortunately, there isn't much choice for kids with flat, wide feet. They need shoes with a wide toe box and maximum arch support and shock absorption. Slip-on loafers aren't right for them.

For more information about childhood foot care, contact your podiatrist.

Chapter 12:

Sports and Your Feet

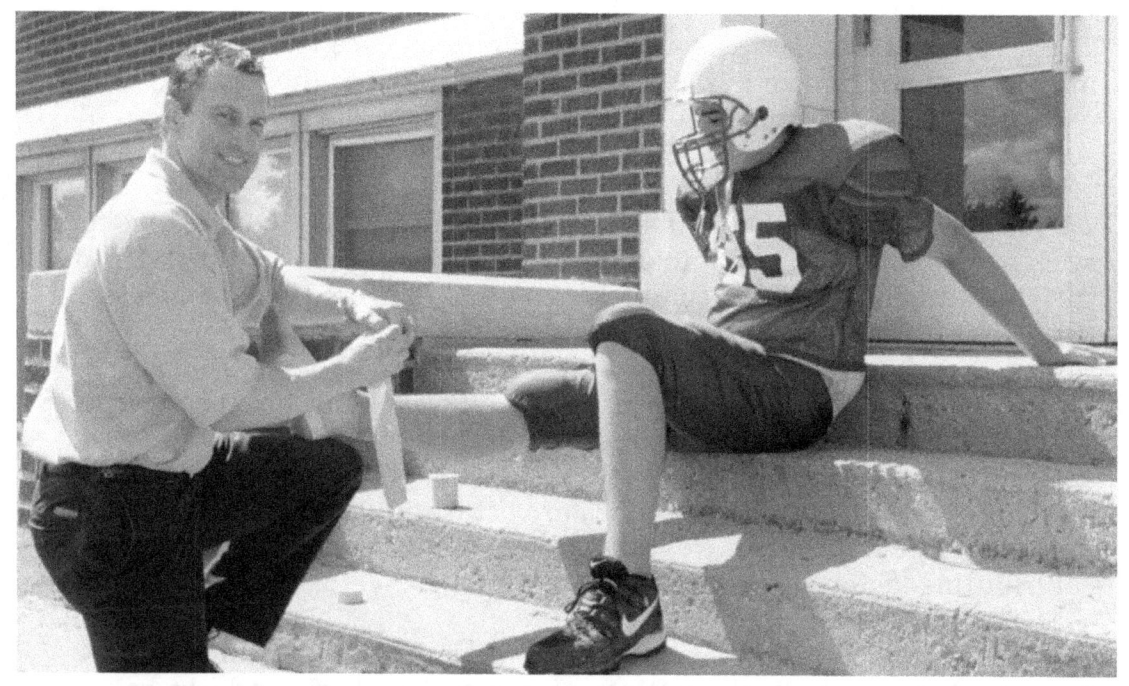

Minnesota Viking's Harrison Smith Sidelined with Turf Toe: Causes & Treatments

Published: *12-21-13*

Football is fun to watch, but it's hard to deny that the sport exposes the body to a variety of foot injuries. A foot injury that is common in football players is turf toe. In fact, Minnesota Vikings safety Harrison Smith limped off the field during the Carolina Panthers games with a left foot injury. He missed the New York Giants game following the injury and is still on the injured reserved list. His foot is healing well, and he is still optimistic he can return this season without needing surgery.

The name sounds funny, but turf toe is no laughing matter to the player who suffers from it. Turf toe is a sprain to the ligaments of the big toe joint. Acting as a pulley for tendons, the sesamoids, two pea-shaped bones located in the ball of the foot, beneath the big-toe joint, help the big toe move normally and provide leverage when the big toe "pushes off" during walking and running.

The sesamoids also serve as a weight-bearing surface for the first metatarsal bone, which is the long bone connected to the big toe, absorbing the weight placed on the ball of the foot when walking, running and jumping.

Turf toe occurs when the big toe is forcibly bent up into hyperextension, such as when pushing off into a sprint while having the toe stuck flat on the ground. This injury is common in football players because artificial turf is harder than natural grass and has less shock absorption.

Turf toe can happen to football players of any level, but also to any sport enthusiast who has increased pressure on the ball of the foot from activities such as running, basketball, football, golf, tennis and ballet. In addition, people with high arches are at risk for developing this problem as well. Frequent wearing of high-heeled shoes can also be a contributing factor.

The most common symptoms of turf toe are pain, swelling and limited movement at the big-toe joint. Symptoms develop slowly and can get worse if there is repeated injury. A forceful injury to the big toe can cause immediate pain that gets worse over 24 hours. Some patients may even feel a pop at the time of injury.

Like ankle sprains, rest, ice, compression and elevation can be used to treat turf toe. If your pain does not resolve or gets worse in the following weeks, you should seek treatment with your podiatrist. If not treated correctly, turf toe can lead to a decrease in the range of motion of the big toe joint and even a complete loss of range of motion.

If you find it difficult to walk on the foot, an x-ray of your foot should be done to rule out a possible fracture. Most turf toe injuries are treated without surgery.

Most turf toe injuries heal within two to three weeks. Physical therapy may be needed for strengthening and range of motion improvement.

Remember to give your toe time to heal. Many of the athletes I treat return to the field too soon, leading to further damage and possibly arthritic changes down the road.

Shin Splints...your Feet May be the Culprit!

Published: 4-20-13

If you are an avid walker, have begun a new exercise program, or are an experienced runner, you may have experienced one of the most common lower extremity ailments, shin splints.

Shin splints are characterized as pain at the front inside area of the shin bone due to over exertion of the muscles. Shin splints usually involve small tears in the leg muscles where they are attached to the shin bone.

The most common cause of shin splints is inflammation of the periostium of the tibia (sheath surrounding the bones). Some other common causes include flat feet (overpronation), a high arch (underpronation), inadequate footwear, running on hard surfaces and increasing training too quickly.

If you have flat feet or a high arch, I always recommend to my patients custom orthotics so that the foot will be supported and align in the neutral position, the correct position for walking and any athletic activity.

Orthotics, also known as orthoses, refers to any device inserted into a shoe, ranging from felt pads to custom-made shoe inserts that correct an abnormal or irregular walking pattern. Sometimes called arch supports, orthotics allow people to stand, walk and run more efficiently and comfortably. While over-the-counter orthotics are available and may help people with mild symptoms, they normally cannot correct the wide range of symptoms that prescription foot orthoses can since they are not custom made to fit an individual's foot structure. So remember, for long term control of your foot condition, you must get a custom orthotic, not an over-the-counter product.

Orthotic devices come in many shapes, sizes and materials and are not the bulky orthotics of the past, so, women, don't be concerned. One must realize though that orthotics will only help after foot inflammation and pain have subsided. Once your foot ailment is relieved, then orthotics can do their job and support your feet without exasperating the issue.

I see many patients wearing inadequate footwear, especially the wrong size. Most people's feet change as they get older and require a different size shoe.

Don't expect the shoes you bought in your 20's to fit in your 40's! This can be hard for women who have invested in a closet full of expensive designer shoes, but better to save your feet now from the worries of corrective surgeries in the future that can have many complications.

Have your feet professionally measured to ensure you have not only the correct length but width in your shoes. This will prevent a host of foot problems down the road.

Use the following tips to treat and prevent shin splints:

For immediate pain relief:
- Ice the area to reduce pain and inflammation.
- Take an over-the-counter anti-inflammatory, like ibuprofen.

For ongoing pain relief:

- Rest to allow the injury to heal.
- Stretch and strengthen the leg muscles.
- Wear insoles or custom orthotics that offer arch support.
- Make sure you have the right running shoe for your foot type and for the activity.
- Avoid running on hard surfaces.
- Shorten your stride.

Consult a podiatrist if your pain is really bad. You should get a full diagnosis to find out if there is a stress fracture in the area.

Bowling and Your Feet

Published: *11-12-11*

When it comes to a sport that provides lots of family fun, few can match a trip to the bowling alley. More than 50 million people go bowling each year.

Most people consider bowling an injury-free sport, but injuries do occur, and stress and strain on the feet can lead to problems throughout the body. The repetitive slide with each throw in bowling is the main cause for added pressure on your feet and it can cause injury if done improperly.

Foot injuries are a lot like back injuries in that they cause a lot of pain during routine tasks that are normally taken for granted. Injuries can be caused by going into the slide wrong and twisting too much, which puts a lot of torque on the leg. This is especially true if your slide foot is angled to the right while you are trying to slide straight. This can cause strain and sprain in the ankle, and repetitive abuse can cause stress fractures.

Bowling shoes are the most overlooked piece of bowling equipment. Many bowlers just don't realize the importance of a good-quality and comfortably fitting bowling shoe.

The left and right bowling shoes offer subtle differences with one being used for sliding and the opposite foot for braking. These varying pressures on different parts of the foot can cause irritations such as blisters and calluses, or even Morton's neuroma, which can be quite painful.

A proper and consistent slide is very important in the execution of a good bowling shot. The athletic or tennis shoe-style bowling shoe is made with a "sliding sole" on both shoes to accommodate left or right handed bowlers. These are considered to be entry-level shoes and an excellent choice for beginners or for bowlers who bowl once a week or less.

The other shoe has rubber on it to assist the bowler in a strong and stable "push off" into the slide. This type of shoe is recommended for bowlers that want to improve their game and for bowlers who bowl more than once a week.

The competitive style shoes are sold with replacement heels and soles for the sliding foot to allow a bowler to adjust their slide distance by changing the slide sole and/or the heel pad on the sliding foot. Therefore, if a bowler is having problems with their slide on a certain approach condition, this shoe will allow the bowler the ability to conquer that issue. They are designed to be worn several times per week. These shoes definitely provide more support at the foul line due to the broader base and firmer fit around the ankle.

Proper footwear and also arch support is critical in bowling, which is why I recommend custom-molded orthotics with your bowling shoes. With custom-molded orthotics, the arch will be supported and take pressure off the joints. They will feel like a part of the shoe and be designed specifically for your foot.

With the latest high-tech materials, such as dual-layered memory foam, custom molded orthotics provide maximum shock absorption without taking up a lot of room in the shoe. You also want to make sure that the top covers are resistant to bacteria, mold and fungus.

Wearing a good set of bowling insoles will not only provide shock absorption, it will also prevent fatigue and improve the bowler's foot comfort. A good set of bowling insoles can also help improve a bowler's coordination which can improve their approach and their scores.

Remember to always prepare for your bowling game by doing a good stretching routine of "toe raises" and "step drop." Bowling is a fun sport. The proper shoes and insoles will provide better coordination and comfort and keep you injury free

Improve Your Golf Swing by Starting with Your Feet

Published: 7-23-11

If your feet aren't in top condition, your golf swing won't be either.

The barrier to a perfect golf swing could lie in your big toe, your heel or the ball of your foot, the three areas of your feet most likely to cause pain that can ruin your golf swing.

Behind these pain-prone spots can be stiff joints, stretched-out tissues and even nerve damage. However, pain relief is possible and usually does not require surgery.

So what are the three most common painful foot conditions that golfers deal with?

The first is heel pain, which typically results from an inflammation of the band of tissue that extends from your heel to the ball of your foot. Heel pain can make it uncomfortable for golfers to maintain a solid stance during crucial portions of their golf swing. People with this condition often compare the pain to someone jabbing a knife in their heel.

The second is arthritis, which causes pain in the joint of your big toe. It can make your golf swing's follow-through difficult.

Finally, neuromas are nerves that become thickened, enlarged and painful because they've been compressed or irritated.

During your golf swing, a neuroma in the ball of your foot can cause significant pain when your body transfers its weight from one foot to the other.

So what's a golfer to do?

If you experience pain while golfing, keep these items in your golf bag to get you through the game:

- A good pain-relief roll-on gel.
- A ball-of-foot gel cushion.
- A gel heel cup for inside your shoes.

Other painful conditions can also cause instability during your swing. Some athletes and former athletes develop chronic ankle instability from previous ankle sprains that failed to heal properly.

Motion-limiting arthritis and Achilles tendonitis can also affect your balance. Ill-fitting golf shoes may cause corns and calluses that make standing uncomfortable.

For the majority of golfers and other patients, I recommend simple treatments such as custom shoe inserts, stretching exercises, changing shoe size, medications, braces, steroid injections or physical therapy.

However, if these conservative measures fail to provide adequate relief, surgery may be required.

Foot pain is not normal, especially when golfing. With the treatment options available to your foot and ankle surgeon today, a pain-free golf swing is clearly in view.

Chapter 13

Women's Foot Health

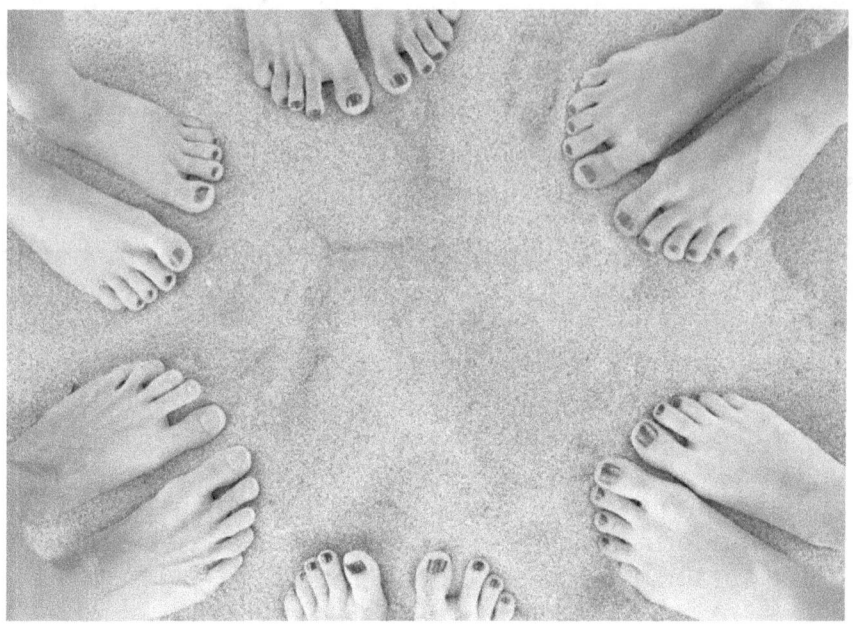

June Brides see Podiatrists in July for Foot Problems

Published: 6-1-13

If June is for brides, then July is certainly for podiatrists, who see brides with foot problems ranging from heel pain to ingrown toenails to the dreaded fungal nail. A pointy, high heeled shoe can cause damage to your feet in just one day.

Sparkles, spangles and color, new or vintage, whatever a new bride's preference in wedding shoe styles, there's one trend that every bride should get behind: comfort. Pretty flats and even tennis shoes have been gaining popularity among brides for several years and, while those styles may not be to everyone's taste, the concept of comfortable wedding shoes is good for everyone.

A recent American Podiatric Medical Association survey indicated that most women do emphasize comfort over looks when choosing dress shoes, but many brides consider comfort less important than style on their big day. Brides may think that, since they're only wearing their wedding shoes for a day, it doesn't matter if the shoes make their feet hurt. But shoes that hurt your feet can cause long term problems, and make existing ones even worse. Not to mention that sore feet can put a damper on your wedding, reception and even the honeymoon.

The trauma of your toes being cramped in a pointy-toed shoe can cause injury to your nail plate and root in just a few hours. This nail can then eventually be susceptible to fungus. And, once you have fungus, it is very difficult to eliminate. Treatment regimens for toenail fungus can last from six months to a year and sometimes can include combinations of topical, oral and laser treatments. Because of the difficulty to break-the-cycle of infection with fungus infections it requires dedication to daily treatments and sanitizing of shoes.

Brides can prevent fungal nail infections by taking these simple precautions, especially on their honeymoon:

- Keep your feet clean and dry.
- Wear shower shoes in public facilities whenever possible.
- Clip nails straight across so that the nail does not extend beyond the tip of the toe.
- Use a quality foot powder (talcum, not cornstarch) in conjunction with shoes that fit well and are made of materials that breathe.
- Avoid wearing excessively tight hosiery, which promotes moisture.
- Socks made of synthetic fiber tend to "wick" away moisture faster than cotton or wool socks, especially for those with more active lifestyles. Try Nano bamboo fiber socks.
- Disinfect home pedicure tools and don't apply polish to nails suspected of infection.

I often see brides with heel pain or plantar fasciitis. The strain that high heels put on the ball of the foot contributes to inflammation in the plantar fascia tendon along the arch of the foot. Often, heel spurs are seen in conjunction with this and sometimes a Haglund's deformity, which is a bump on the back of the heel.

Treatments today for plantar fasciitis no longer involve surgery, in most cases. Exercises, custom orthotics and stretching of the tendon often help and are the first course for treatment.

In the rare instance that these fail, I always recommend shockwave therapy and/or autogolous blood platelet injections before jumping into surgery. Most women don't want the complications of surgery which can be numerous including months of recovery with non-weight bearing, infection and swelling at the surgical site. I always consider surgery for plantar fasciitis and heel spurs a last resort.

When a bride calls my office after coming back from her honeymoon, I know it was from wearing the wrong type or size shoes. I often get a call that the big toe is red, painful and swollen. This is the tell-tale sign of an ingrown toenail. Although most ingrown toenails are due to the curvature of your toenail, wearing the wrong size shoe can cramp your toes and cause the nail border to start to grow inward into the skin. This can be very painful.

Ingrown toenails start out hard, swollen and tender. Left untreated, they may become sore, red, and infected and the skin may start to grow over the ingrown toenail.

In most cases, treating ingrown toenails is simple: Soak the foot in warm, soapy water several times each day. Avoid wearing tight shoes or socks. Antibiotics are sometimes prescribed if an infection is present.

Note: Please consult your physician before taking any medications.
In severe cases, if an acute infection occurs, surgical removal of part of the ingrown toenail may be needed. Known as partial nail plate avulsion, the procedure involves injecting the toe with an anesthetic and cutting out the ingrown part of the toenail.

So for all those June brides: choose comfort over style with shoes and avoid a visit in July to your podiatrist.

Female Athletes at Risk for Foot & Ankle Injuries During Menstrual Cycle

Published: *3-24-12*

Research at the University of Melbourne has found that women's menstrual cycles can increase their risk of injuries, but those who take contraceptive pills are more likely to be protected. Injuries of the foot and ankle are significantly heightened at the beginning and middle of a women's cycle.

At the beginning, there is reduced muscle tone and coordination due to lower estrogen levels. On day 14 of the cycle, estrogen levels are at their peak and this increases the elasticity of the Achilles tendon and the risk of injury.

The most common Achilles tendon injuries are Achilles tendinosis, or tendonitis, and Achilles tendon rupture.

Achilles tendon ruptures, also known as tears, can be full ruptures or partial ruptures.

Achilles tendinosis, which is also known as Achilles tendinopathy, is soreness and stiffness that comes on gradually and continues to worsen until treated. It is a common injury among middle- and long-distance runners.

The severity of Achilles tendinosis can be broken down into four grades which can be measured in terms of how the Achilles tendon feels during exercise, the amount of stiffness and creaking, and the Achilles tendon's soreness to the touch.

The four grades are:

1. No pain during exercise, but there is some discomfort in the morning when first getting out of bed. The stiffness and creaking go away after a few minutes and are fine the rest of the day. Lightly pinching the Achilles tendon with the forefinger and thumb in the morning or after exercise will probably indicate soreness.
2. Pain during exercise or running, but performance is not affected. The stiffness and creaking appear when first getting out of bed and disappear shortly afterward. Lightly pinching the Achilles tendon with the forefinger and thumb in the morning or after exercise will indicate soreness.
3. Pain during exercise or running that is detrimental to performance. The stiffness and creaking appear when first getting out of bed and may continue for some time and reappear at other points during the day. Lightly pinching the Achilles tendon with the forefinger and thumb in the morning or after exercise will indicate soreness.
4. Pain is too great to exercise or run. The stiffness and creaking appear when first getting out of bed and may continue for most of the day. Lightly pinching the Achilles tendon with the forefinger and thumb at almost any time of day will indicate soreness.

The researchers at the University of Melbourne, however, have found that women who take contraceptive pills have lower injury rates because the pill reduces the level of circulating estrogen.

Elite female athletes may consider taking the contraceptive pill or hormone replacement therapy to reduce the risk of injury.

Research has shown women become more prone to injury when they train at an elite level. This is because they over-train and under-eat. This causes their estrogen levels to fluctuate more than usual.

In light of this evidence, women who exercise regularly and intensely should take extra precaution during their menstrual cycle by wearing shoes that support their feet and ankles. Women athletes who train daily should see their podiatrist if they have any Achilles tendon problems.

Enjoy Pregnancy without Foot Pain

Published: *3-20-10*

"Oh, my aching feet!" is a phrase you often hear from pregnant women.

However, sore feet are not just a symptom for women during pregnancy.

Women often experience foot pain during pregnancy because of increased weight, foot instability and swelling. In the last five years, I have seen an increase in pregnant women with foot pain because women are more active than ever before, even running marathons during their pregnancies.

I recommend the following guidelines to help reduce foot pain during pregnancy.

Pregnant women often experience throbbing, swollen feet due to excess fluid build up, or edema, in their feet from the weight and position of the baby. To reduce swelling, put your feet up whenever possible, stretch your legs frequently, wear wide comfortable shoes, and avoid crossing your legs when sitting.

Pain in the arch can be due to arch fatigue or overpronation, also known as flattening of the arch. Overpronation occurs due to extreme stress to the ligament that holds up the arch of the foot. The best way to prevent arch pain is to stretch in the morning and before and after any exercise. Also, do not go barefoot and make sure to wear supportive, low-heeled shoes.

Foot cramps are caused by increased blood volume and high progesterone levels brought on by pregnancy. To prevent cramps, increase circulation by rotating ankles and elevating feet while sitting.

If cramps persist, try a walk around the block and stretch your calf muscles every day.

Painful, ingrown toenails can be caused by excessive stress from tight-fitting shoes. Give your feet a break by wearing wider shoes during the last trimester of pregnancy. If you have an ingrown toenail, avoid attempting "bathroom surgery." Repeated cutting of the nail can cause the condition to worsen over time. It is best to seek treatment with a foot and ankle surgeon.

Believe it or not, it is common for women to experience a change in their foot size during pregnancy. A permanent growth of up to half a size in women's feet can occur from the release of a hormone called relaxin; the same hormone that allows the pelvis to open to deliver the baby. Relaxin makes the ligaments in your feet more flexible, causing feet to spread wider and longer.

Pregnancy and pending motherhood should be a joy. If foot pain persists, a podiatrist can provide relief with conservative treatments like physical therapy, foot orthotics, supportive shoes and minor toenail procedures.

Bunions in Women's Feet Worse in Fall Boots

Published: *10-3-09*

Fall is often a painful time for many women. As women transition from open-toed sandals to closed-in boots and shoes, more of them seek relief for painful bunions. This trend plays out every fall. Some female bunion patients are in agony and describe a constant, throbbing pain, even when they take their shoes off.

A bunion is a bone deformity caused by an enlargement of the joint at the base and side of the big toe. Bunions form when the toe moves out of place. The enlargement then causes more irritation or swelling. In some cases, the big toe moves toward the second toe and rotates or twists. Bunions can also lead to other toe deformities, such as hammertoes.

It is estimated that 33 percent of the population in Western countries suffer from bunions. Bunions are often inherited and tend to run in families, usually because of a faulty foot structure. Foot injuries, neuromuscular problems, flat feet and pronated feet can also contribute to their formation.

Wearing shoes that are too tight can aggravate bunions, as many women with bunions suffer from discomfort and pain from the constant irritation, rubbing and friction of the enlargement against shoes.

The skin over the toe becomes red and tender, and because this joint flexes with every step, the bigger the bunion gets, the more it hurts to walk.

Over time, bursitis or arthritis may set in, the skin on the bottom of the foot may become thicker, and walking may become difficult, all contributing to chronic pain.

Some women ask about bunion surgery in the fall because they're less busy than in the summer months. Also, many are closer to meeting their insurance deductibles. Surgery is a last resort treatment for painful bunions. In many cases, simple changes like wearing shoes with wider toe boxes can reduce bunion pain.

Custom shoe inserts, gel or foam-filled padding and anti-inflammatory medications may also provide pain relief. When the pain of a bunion interferes with a woman's daily activities, then it's time to discuss surgical options. Depending on the size of the enlargement, misalignment of the toe, and level of pain, different surgery techniques may be advised to remove the bunion and realign the toe.

The sooner you see your podiatrist to discuss treatment options, the sooner you'll be on the road to enjoying life's activities again.

Chapter 14
Bonus Section

Findlay Footsteps- Courier Article

Shoe Recommendations

How to Choose an Athletic Shoe

Stretching Exercises

Buy Book at 20% OFF on Amazon with coupon code: 6USG7XSK

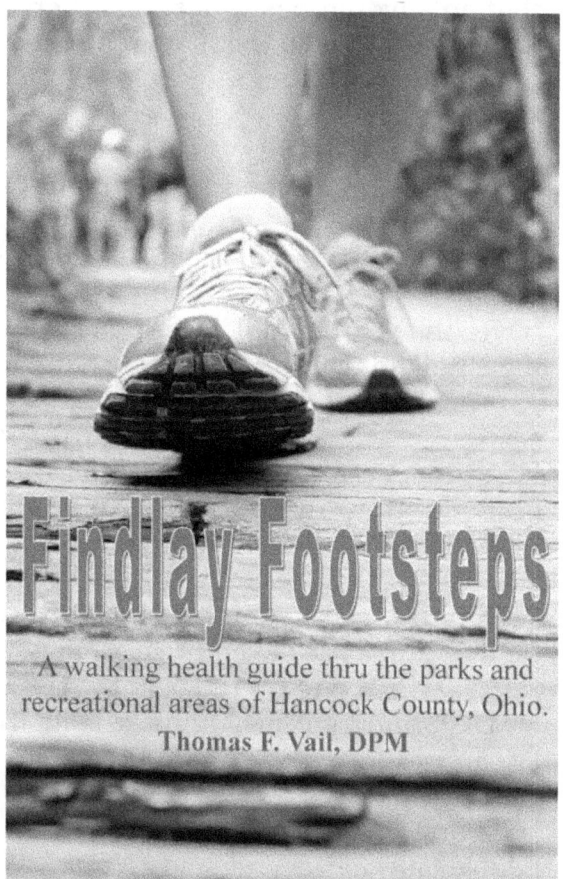

Lace Up and Get Fit

Published: *10-18-12*

Podiatrist publishes area walking guide

By JEANNIE WILEY WOLF STAFF WRITER 'The Courier'

Dr. Thomas F. Vail believes one of the best prescriptions for a healthier lifestyle is walking.

So the Findlay podiatrist has developed "Findlay Footsteps," a pictorial guide of walking paths, bike trails and outdoor activities in Findlay and surrounding areas. The book is designed to show people that exercising is as easy as walking around a local park.

"This got started on our blog (Findlay Foot Facts)," said Vail, who has practiced in Findlay for over 20 years.

"Patients would post questions there about how to exercise, what they could do, and walking is a great exercise so we tried to think of places they could go," he said.

"And then I thought, well, there should be a little pictorial book of all the places in Findlay that people might not know about."

Office manager Joe Yorey also got on board with the project.

"Over the years people would come to us and say, it would be really nice if we had some kind of book based on that blog, so that's what kind of got us into the idea of doing this," he said.

Yorey helped with organization of the information, and Jackie Faeth, a student intern in Vail's office, took the photographs that appear in the book. Some foot facts are included as well.

Vail himself works out on an elliptical machine during the week. But if he has time on weekends, he enjoys walking at Riverside Park, Riverbend Recreation Area and the Findlay reservoirs. Vail also likes to rollerblade on the Slippery Elm Trail that runs from North Baltimore to Bowling Green.

"Walking is one of the best exercises because it is low-impact and most people can do it," Vail said. "You're not going to stress and strain with the knees and the hips, and it's inexpensive. Can't afford a membership to the Y? You can walk."

"Get outside and exercise. Keep that cholesterol down. Diabetics, keep their sugar down. Everybody can do it," he said.

Yorey said the book took six to eight months to compile. "We go through parks, but not just parks," he said. "We go through walking downtown, the Cube. We have a lot of things in there that are not just outside, walking in the mall, their backyard, walking around their neighborhood."

Also included are some of the special events unique to Findlay such as KidsFest, Flag City Balloon Fest and the Riverside Summer Concert Series.

"When you start to look at all the stuff that's going on in Findlay and where you can go and do these things, it's pretty amazing," Vail said.

He noted that one of the major problems people encounter when they begin an exercise program is not knowing what type of shoes to buy or how they should fit.

"The biggest problem we see is shoe fit," Vail said. "It's usually the wrong size, the wrong fit." "To get the proper fit, go one finger beyond your longest toe.

Some people have that long dominant second toe, so you want to make sure it's one finger beyond that toe. And then the width, just make sure it's a little bit snug but not too tight," he said.

Vail said shoes that are too small can lead to toenail fungus.

"A lot of it is people's fit and mostly women because your shoes are tapered, and the high heel shoes put a lot of pressure and that lets the little fungus and spores in," he said. "Once we get the shoes then treat the fungus, you have a good chance of it not coming back."

Another tip, he said, is to go shoe shopping late in the afternoon. Feet swell later in the day.

"And we don't walk in pumps, high heels, or sandals and flip flops, lots of injuries with those," Vail said. "We usually prefer a tie, lace-up shoe."

"Some of the Velcro shoes are OK for those that have arthritis and can't tie, but slip-ons and flip flops and things like that aren't structurally sound for walking, so stay away from those," he said.

Get a good shoe fit, he said, and you can go out and do these things.

"So many patients come in here and say they can't exercise because their feet hurt, and a lot of times we find out that it basically is they didn't have the right shoe," Yorey added.

Vail noted that stretching before a walk or any kind of exercise is also important. "Walking up and down steep hillsides and tramping through wet, slippery fields and wooded areas puts stress on the muscles and tendons in the feet and ankles, especially if you haven't conditioned properly before hitting the trail," he said. "Also many people don't realize that cross-training athletic shoes aren't the best choice for extended hiking trails. Had some of my patients worn a sturdy, well-constructed shoe they wouldn't have suffered sprained ankles or strained Achilles tendons." Stretching will also help people who have planter fasciitis or heel spurs, Vail said. "Sometimes we have to augment the good shoe with a little bit of an arch orthotic support in there to help alleviate that, but stretching does a great job in helping alleviate that pain," he said.

And the right socks can help prevent blisters. Vail recommended synthetic socks that have moisture wicking properties and nano bamboo charcoal fibers which are anti-microbial.

He also noted that pain can occur from overuse, even from walking. "If you're not accustomed to walking on sloped or uneven ground your legs and feet will get tired and cause muscles and tendons to ache," he said. "To avoid a serious injury, such as a severe ankle sprain or an Achilles tendon rupture, rest for a while if you start hurting. Serious injury risk escalates significantly if you continue walking in pain." Beginners should take on less difficult trails until they become better conditioned and more confident, Vail said.

The book can be purchased on Amazon for $17.99. Hancock County Residents can us Coupon Code 6USG7XSK to get a 20% discount. For anyone who would like to see the book before they order, copies are available at Vail's Office at 1725 Western Ave., Suite C.

Top Pediatric Shoes

The following children's shoes are given my 'top' recommendation for both functionality and comfort:

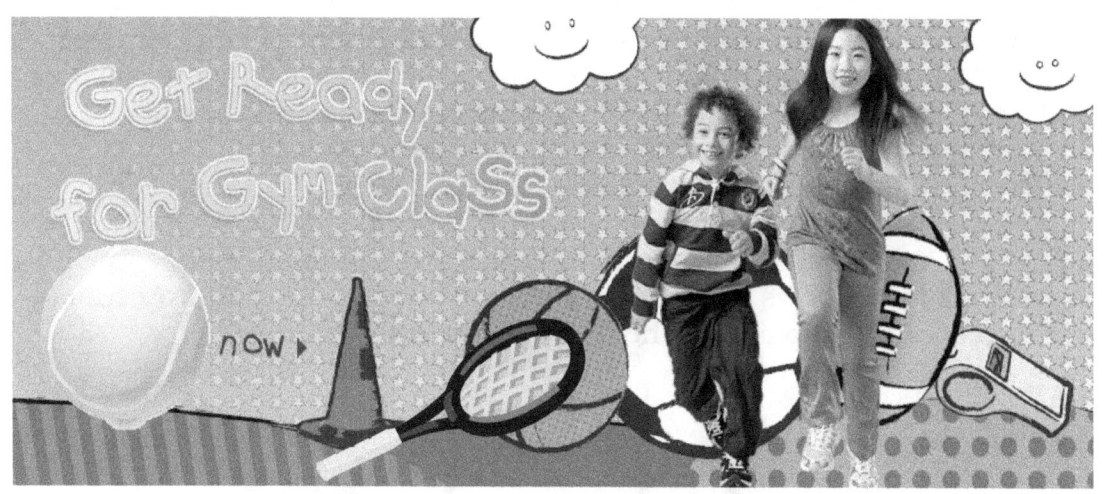

ASICS America Corporation

Young runners and athletes will receive superior cushioning and durability in the performance oriented Asics line of athletic shoes. Features of Asics athletic shoes include GEL® Cushioning System, the lightweight stability of the Trusstic System®, airmesh upper, and durable reinforced stitched toe caps.

My Recommendations: Gel-Nimbus 12 GS, Gel-1160 GS, Gel-Cumulus 12 GS, Gel-Trabuco 13 GS, Gel-160 TR GS, GT-2150 GS

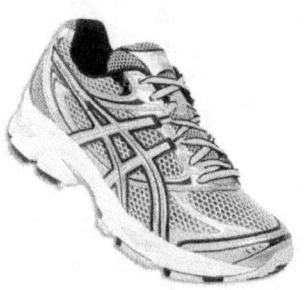

Gel-Cumulus 12 GS

Pediped™ Footwear
Pediped™ Footwear: All lines especially the Originals and Flex.

Officially recognized by the American Podiatric Medical Association as contributing to better foot health, Pediped™ footwear is a smart choice for parents concerned with the long-term development of children's feet. Pediped™ has been awarded the prestigious APMA seal of acceptance for both it's Originals and Flex lines in support of their many beneficial attributes that promote quality foot health including soft cushioned leather soles, a wide toe box and soft leather uppers.

As babies' and toddlers' feet begin to develop, a soft, pliable shoe, such as pediped footwear, is essential to not only provide the foot protection, but also enough mobility for the foot to properly form.

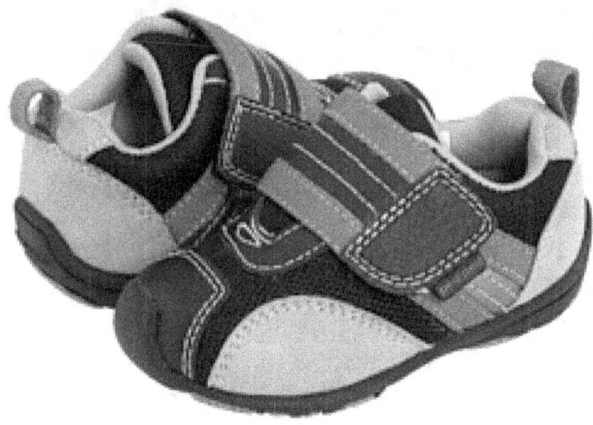

Pediped™ Adrian

Reebok

These Reebok athletic shoes have low-cut designs for increased stability, synthetic/mesh uppers for comfort, support and breathability, forefoot flexibility and air cushioning for comfort.

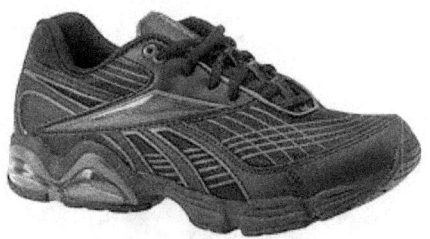

Reebok Flash-Alac

My Recommendations: Flash-Alac, Motion Lace (Grade School), Bet on this Laces (Grade School/Pre-School), Wind Magic II (Grade School/Pre-School), Back to It Lace (Grade School/ Pre-School), Wind Magic Lace (Grade School/Pre-School), FlexRide Road III

Brooks
Brooks offers neutral shoes for very small children and more supportive shoes for kids who overpronate.

My Recommendations:
Little Kid/Big Kid Defyance Sneaker, Kids Adrenaline GTS, Kids Ghost Defyance Kids Sneaker

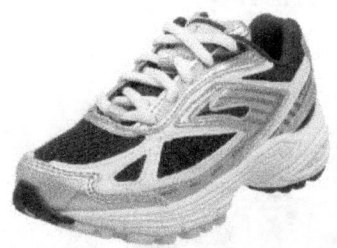

New Balance

At New Balance not all shoes are created equal! New youth sizing accommodates all kids' sizes from toddler to teen and they have shoes specifically designed for infants, pre-school and Grade school.

My Recommendations: Style 631 (infants), Style 687 (Pre-school), and Style 759 (Grade School)

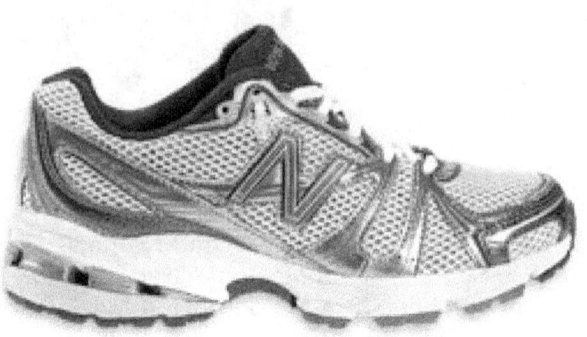

Adidas

Adidas athletic shoes have air mesh uppers for maximum ventilation, textile lining and EVA insole for comfort , TORSION® SYSTEM for midfoot integrity; adiPRENE®+ in the forefoot to maintain propulsion and efficiency, and adiPRENE® under the heel for superior cushioning at impact.

Our Recommendations: Supernova Sequence, Supernova Glide X XTD, Adilastic Bounce and the Hyperrun 3

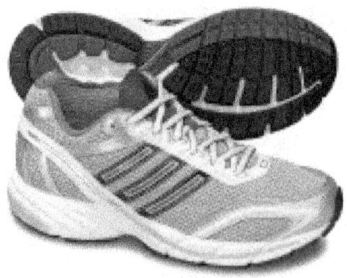

Supernova Glide X XTD

Robeez by Stride-Rite - Baby Shoes

The best shoe mimics bare feet, by supporting - not constricting tiny growing feet. Robeez footwear flex and bend with every step. They promote good balance and unrestricted growth, while protecting little feet from the world. They stay on too, with elasticized ankles to ensure a perfectly snug fit. From crawling to cruising, walking to running, for indoors and out, Robeez makes different shoes for newborns to four-year-olds.

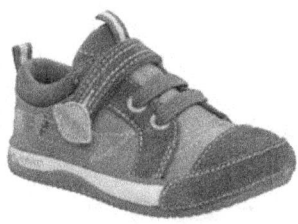

Robeez 1st Stepz

My Recommendations: Robeez Luxury Soft Sole Collection, Robeez Mini Shoez Collection, Robeez Soft Soles and Bootie, Robeez 1st Stepz, Robeez Eco Collection

See Kai Run

The advantages to See Kai Run shoes are many! While podiatrists and pediatricians now agree that barefoot is best for proper foot and muscular development, it is not always practical. Flexible soles are recommended because they are protective for indoor and outdoor wear, yet not restrictive. The soles of See Kai Run Smaller booties are made from soft suede, with non-slip rubber pads for traction. 'See Kai Run' shoes incorporate a very flexible, yet durable rubber for the soles of first walkers. Both allow plenty of freedom for developing little feet.

My Recommendations: See Kai Run Children's soft booties, See Kai Run Children's First Walkers, Eleven by See Kai Run for bigger kids.

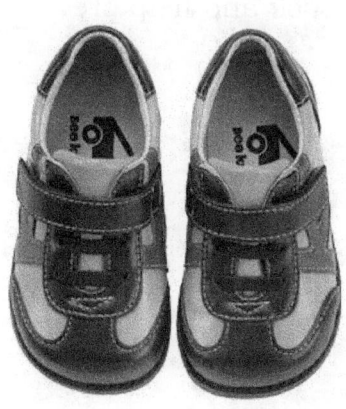

Here are two great companies for Kids insoles and socks!

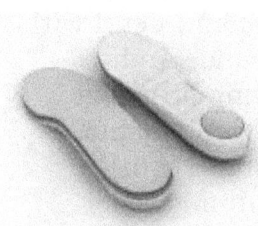

Spenco: Kids Polysorb Insoles

Today's active kids need foot support and cushioning that's designed for growing feet. After the age of five, when the bones, muscles and ligaments of the foot begin to fully develop, Spenco Kids® Insoles (along with quality shoes and pediatric care) are an important part of a kid's foot future.

Spenco Kids Polysorb Insoles

SmartKnit KIDS Seamless Socks

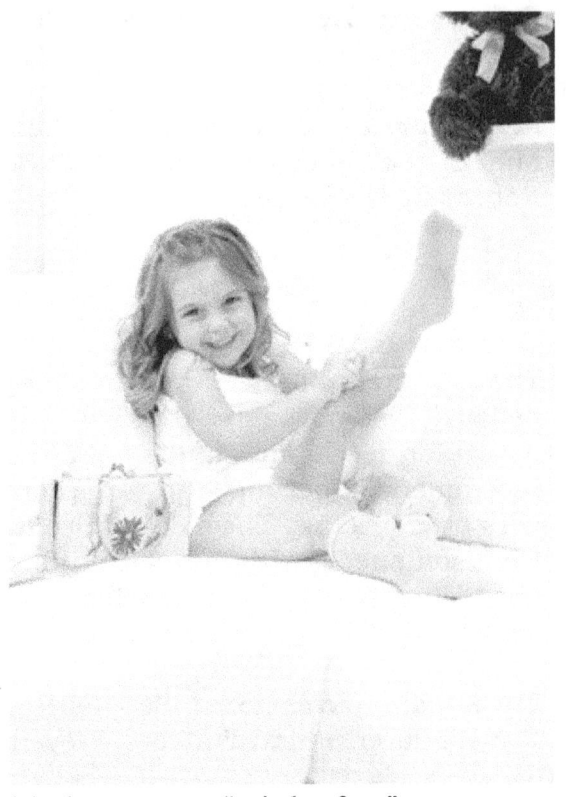

SmartKnit Kids Socks are completely free of seams providing comfort and relief to children who struggle with "bumps & lumps" in their socks. They also feature a non-binding Halo Top™ that fits comfortably without slipping down the leg. Regular socks often have elastic bands at the tops of the sock that can often pinch, bind or be a source of irritation. Lastly, high-tech fibers wick moisture away helping ensure a drier sock and help prevent "stinky feet".

Adult Shoe Recommendations

This recommended shoe list compiles many of the best shoes that I have found. For the most part they are shoes that offer increased stability. For most people with foot problems, a stable shoe allows the foot to function in a more normal manner and helps the foot perform its natural job of absorbing shock. Of course, this is a generalized list and your needs may be somewhat different.

The buyer must be aware that due to the frequently changing styles and product numbers in the shoe industry a list of manufacturers and style 'group' is not always current. A list of shoe manufacturers and their websites is included. Please consult the appropriate web-sites for each manufacturer to locate a specific style for your individual needs. Please be advised to look for shoes that offer the most stability not motion.

Shoe Manufacturer Websites:

- *Nike Air*
  www.nike.com
- *Rockport Pro Walker/Dress Rockport*
  www.rockport.com
- *Reebok Tennis shoes with Air Cushion/Walkers*
  www.reebok.com
- *New Balance*
  www.newbalance.com
- *Avia*
  www.avia.com
- *Easy Spirit Dress Shoes*
  www.easyspirit.com
- *Naturalizer*
  www.naturalizer.com

Work Shoes
- *Red Wing*
  www.redwingshoes.com
- *Mason*
  www.masonezpay.com
- *Wolverine*
  www.wolverine.com

SHOE RECOMMENDATIONS

Shoes on this list have the following features:

Anti-pronation
Torsional Stability
Removable Insole
Firm Heel Counter
Firm Medial Midsole

Exercise Walking/Running

- **New Balance:** 1011*, 587(lat), 817 (rocker sole), 766
- **Asics Gel:** Foundation, 2120, Kayano
- **Etonic:** Stable Pro
- **Nike:** Equalon, Structure Triax
- **Brooks:** Beast*/Ariel*, Addiction, Adrenaline, Vapor
- **Saucony:** Grid Stabil*, Omni, Hurricane
- **Adidas:** Adistar Control, Response Control
- **Mizuno:** Renegade

Walking

- **Rockport:** Pro Walker DMX
- **New Balance:** 926, 811, 757
- **Brooks:** Addiction WT (Leather)
- **Saucony:** Grid Stabil
- **SAS:** Time Out (m), Free Time (w)
- **Aetrex:** X800 and X900 Series

Trail Run/Walking/Light Hiking

- **Merrill:** Chameleon
- **Brooks:** Addiction ASR
- **Montrail:** Hardrock* Hurricane Ridge

Cross Trainers

- **Asics:** Gel-Alta (volleyball, xtrain)
- **Nike:** Air Trainer Huarache, Air Max Trainer (tennis)*
- **New Balance:** 1008, 854, 1002 (tennis)

Basketball

- **Nike Air:** Air Force STAT, Air Huarache, Max Elite
- **Adidas:** KG Bounce, T-MAC
- **NewBalance:** 904, 8026

Sandals

Bite   Naot   Finn Comfor   Dansko   Ariat   Theresia   Kumfs
Crocs Rx: Diabetic Cloud, Relief, Silver Cloud
Birkenstock: Kansas, Nebraska, Sabina, Navarro, Sheridan, Madera

Dress Shoes: Flats, Clogs, Casual

Dress Shoes should fit the following criteria:
- **Firm Heel**
- **Torsionally Stable (do not twist easily)**
- **Removable insole**

The following brands have several models which fit the above criteria. Evaluate the shoes carefully, **not all models fit the criteria.**

Specific Models are not mentioned as dress models change rapidly
Rockport, Hush Puppies, Ariat, Dansko, Kumfs, Wolky, Timberland, Sanita, Nickels, Aravon, Naot, Dunham, Sudini, Selby, Theresia, Munro, Paul Thomas, Neil M, Salamander, Nautica, Natural Step

Extra Depth

Apex, Aetrex, PW Minor, Acor, Sequoia, Orthofeet, Comfortrite, Drew, Pedors (offer stretch for forefoot)

Diabetic Shoes -*Note that these shoes are not only for Diabetics*

but may benefit anyone needing a good supportive Shoe
Natural Step, New Balance Model 811 or 812, Dav-Mar, Dr. Comfort

Slippers

Crocs, Geisswein Clogs, Daniel Green Clogs, Merrill Slides, Stegmann Clogs, Naot Aster or Glacier, Haflinger, Finn Comfort Aussie, Dr. Comfort

Socks-Avoid all cotton socks

Thor-lo, Cool-Max, Smartwool, Pedi-Fix, Jobst(For Diabetics), Juno(For Diabetics), WrightSock, Aetrex-Diabetic Line, Dr. Comfort

Insoles

Spenco Flat Insole-under or over orthotic, Dr. Jill's Pump Pals Gel Insole

Prefabricated Arch Supports (in order of stability)

Powerstep Pro-Tech Fl, 3/4, and Classic, Spenco Orthotic Arch Support & Polysorb

Key Code: *Maximum Control-These models have removable insoles and can accept custom orthoses.

Friendly Footwear For Those Who Work Standing Up!

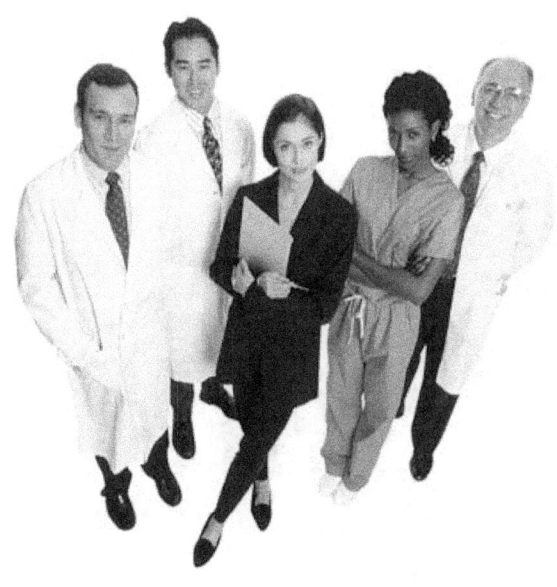

Excessive standing and walking on hard surfaces like concrete increase the incidence of foot problems. However, many footwear companies create products that are specifically made for those who "work standing up."

The following footwear products, designed specifically for those who make a living on their feet, have been granted APMA's Seal of Acceptance.

The Seal of Acceptance Program recognizes products which have been found beneficial to foot health and of significant value when used in a consistently applied program of daily foot care and regular profession treatment.

Crocs Work Shoes

Hover, Bistro, Ginger High Velocity, Saffron, Specialist, Specialist Vent, Velocity

The familiar, comfortable feel of Crocs is also available in a profession-looking shoe that conforms to workplace standards. Featuring a closed toe and heel design, as well as arch support and a foot bed that promotes circulation, the Crocs Work Shoe is a top choice for many health and service industry professionals across the country.

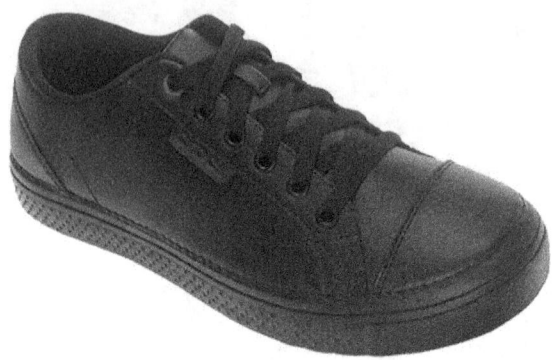

Dansko, LLC

Acadia Collection, Belmont Collection, Sausalito Collection

Dansko's Acadia collection features distressed leather uppers, a removable triple density molded EA insole and slip resistant out-sole. With a light weight base and lower profile, this collection is perfect for the active woman. Additionally, the company's Stapled Collection features a rigid construction and key features that promote good foot health, including a rocker bottom and full arch support.

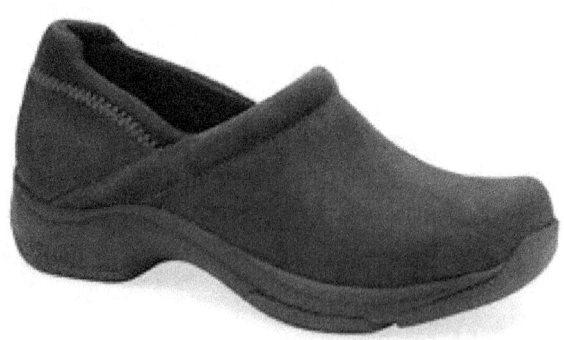

The Timberland Company

Timberland PRO

Timberland's PRO Renova series of work footwear-which includes the Profession, Provider, and Caregiver (pictured) is designed specifically for those at work in the health care community. The Professional Series features Timberland PRO Anti-Fatigue technology, a rocker profile, and an anatomically shaped oblique last for all-day comfort.

Timberland PRO Caregiver Series: (sku#: 65686, 65688, 65689, 65691, 85617), Timberland PRO Professional Series (sku#: 85612, 85613, 85614, 85615, 85616), Timberland PRO Renova Provider Series (sku#:85618, 85619, 65694)

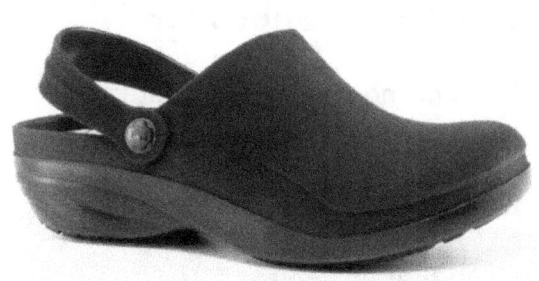

Sanita Clogs, Inc.

Leisure Collection-Safe, Leo Pro-Men's Closed Back Clog, Lisa and Leo Safe-Men's and Women's Safety Clogs w/Steel Toe, Lisa and Leo Safe-Men's and Women's Safety Clogs w/Steel Toe and Cap, Lisa Pro-Women's Closed Back Clog, Vera Pro-Women's Open Back Clog, Viktor Pro-Men's Open Back Clog

Footwear Industries Prty Ltd.

Steel Blue Footwear:

Men's Safety (Stee-toe) Models-Argyle, Bronco, Bundaberg, Cobar, Collie, Eucla, Heeler, Hobart, Jarrah, Karratha, Portland, Riverina, Wagga, Warragul, and Whyalla.

Men's Safety (Steel-toe and Steel Penetration Resistant Midsoles) Models-Argyle, Bronco, Bundaberg, Cobar, Collie, Eucla, Heeler, Hobart, Jarrah, Karratha, Portland, RIverina, Wagga, Warragul, and Whyalla.

Women's Safety (Steel-toe) Models-Amery, Capel, Mallina, Maya, Tammin, and Vivien.

Hy-test Safety Footwear

Hy-Test Footholds® Slip Resistant Footwear, Hy-Test Footrest® Safety Footwear

Nunn Bush

Frank, Williams

The Rockport Company

Rockport Works collection

How to Choose an Athletic Shoe that's Right for You

Selecting the correct shoe for your activity and foot type can go a long way in preventing many foot related injuries and can reduce the risk of accelerating and aggravating many foot deformities. The running community has known this for many years. Indeed many dedicated runners have spent years attempting to find "just the right" shoe that both fits their foot and provides them with the appropriate amount of function and protection to prevent injuries. Acknowledging the high number of miles that we expect our feet to carry us during a lifetime and the cumulative toll these miles extract, it becomes clear that the same type of selection process that a runner uses to select a running shoe should also be applied to the shoes that we wear to and from work, at work and at home each day.

To that end, the following guideline and suggestions may assist you in preventing injury and/or slowing down the progression of foot deformities such that you avoid being tallied in the above statistics.

To begin with, we need to recognize that the foot is an extremely complicated and intricate structure; a collection of bones, joints, ligaments and tendons working in concert to support our body weight over a variety of surface types and provide a mechanism with which to flexibly adapt to these surface during the heel strike portion of the gait cycle and conversely, change into a rigid lever to provide adequate propulsion as you push off with your toes. Many foot related injuries and deformities can occur when these seemingly opposite functions of the foot are not working in the correct proportions. The selection of an appropriate shoe will many times help keep these functions working in a more ideal manner.

Feet come in many different sizes and shapes. For the most part, we can divide these feet into three categories:

1) The low arched straight foot
2) The medium arched slightly curved foot
3) The high arched and usually more curved foot

Fortunately, many running shoes are manufactured on two basic lasts (shape of the overall construction of the shoe) and can usually be divided into three overall functional types. Motion Control shoes are typically based upon a straight last design and are usually suited for people with low arched, straight feet. Stability Type shoes are for those individuals with a medium arched foot (typically deemed "normal") and have a slight curve to the shape of the shoe. Lastly, Neutral Type shoes are based upon a curved last and best fit those individuals with a high arched foot. Additionally, as you examine shoes from each of these categories, you may notice that as you move from a neutral type shoe to a stability type shoe and on to a motion controlling type shoe, the shoes become more rigid and thus more resistant to twisting and bending.

Body weight can factor into the selection process. Increased weight places more demands upon your feet and as such, one might consider increasing the level of protection a shoe can offer by selecting a shoe from a greater controlling category i.e.: opting for a motion control shoe rather than a stability shoe over a neutral shoe. Just remember to make sure the shoe fits comfortably on your foot before you purchase the shoe. Consider trying on shoes near the end of your day when your foot is at its largest. And use the socks or stockings that you intend to use with those particular shoes.

The following are some examples of running type shoes within each category. This list is not meant to be all inclusive, but rather it is intended to be used as a guide to assist you in your selection process. You may consider asking your shoe retailer for additional assistance.

Neutral Shoes for the High Arched Foot:

Adidas: Supernova Cushion or Supernova Classic
Asics: Nimbus or Cumulus
Brooks: Glycerin, Dyad, or Epiphany
Mizuno: Wave Creation 5 or Wave Rider 7
New Balance: 1022 or 880
Nike: Pegasus
Pearl Izumi: VisIQ
Saucony: Trigon Responsive

Stability Shoes for the Medium Arched Foot:

Adidas: Supernova Control
Asics: Gel-Kayano 10, Creed, GT 2090, or Gel 1090
Brooks: Trance, Adrenaline GTS 5, or Vantage
Mizuno: Alchemy or Wave Mercury 4
New Balance: 991, 855, 765, or 716
Nike: Structure Triax, Moto, or Althea
Saucony: Hurricane or Omni

Motion Control Shoes for the Low Arched Foot:

Adidas: Brevard or Cairo
Asics: Gel Foundation Plus
Brooks: Ariel or Addiction
Etonic: Pro3 MC2
Mizuno: Legend or Renegade
New Balance: 587
Nike: Durham
Saucony: Stabil MC

Foot and Ankle Exercises

1. Wall Push Up: Stand up straight about three feet from a wall. Ensure that you are facing the wall. Lean forward and place your hands on the wall; bend your arms at your elbows. Keep legs straight, knees locked, feet flat with toes pointed inward. Hold for 10 seconds. Relax. Repeat 6 times.

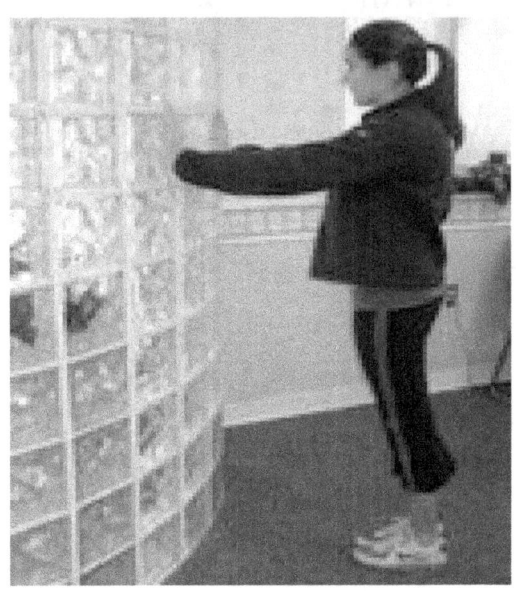

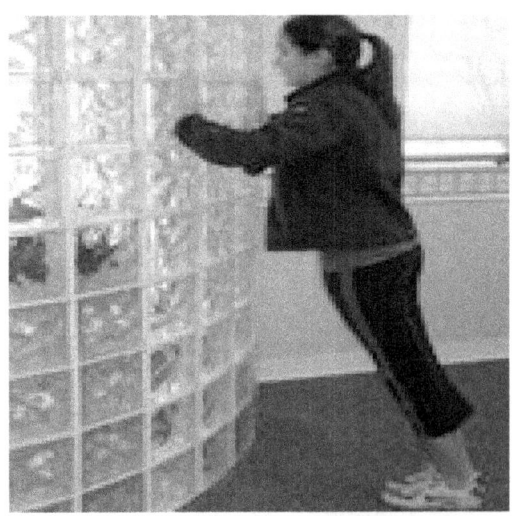

2. Hamstring Stretch: Standing up, place one foot onto a small stool. Keep your leg straight and your knees locked. Once in this position bring your head toward the knee of the leg that is on the stool. Hold this position for 30 seconds and then relax. Repeat 6 times for each leg. You may gradually work to a higher position by increasing the height of the stool.

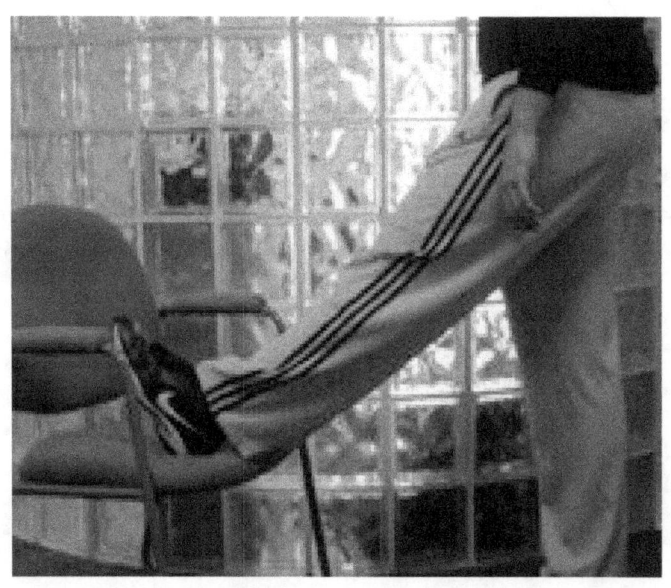

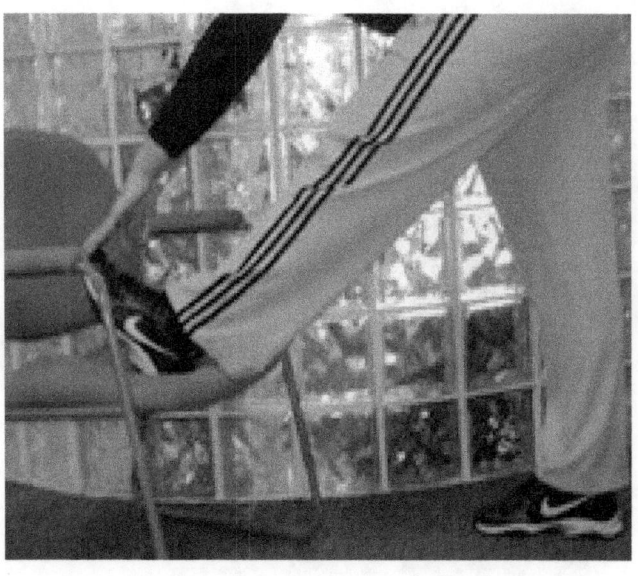

3. **Eccentric Exercise for Plantar Fasciitis:** Directions:
   - Standing on an elevated surface or a slant board, bend the left knee so that it is parallel to the floor. This knee should be bent and flexed. Drop the heel down on the right leg. Raise the right heel to neutral and then drop down. Repeat for opposite extremity. Do this with the knee extended and flexed as shown in photos.
   - This exercise should be done to 'fatigue' but not create increased pain. Gradually add weight to a backpack in .5 lb increments every 4 days as your strength and pain endurance increases.
   - It is *very important* to add weight slowly as it can make the difference between having success or failure. (Soup Cans work nicely!)
   - Do three sets of fifteen reps two times per day for twelve weeks
   - It is very important to keep a daily log book including the number of repetitions, the amount of weight used and a pain score.

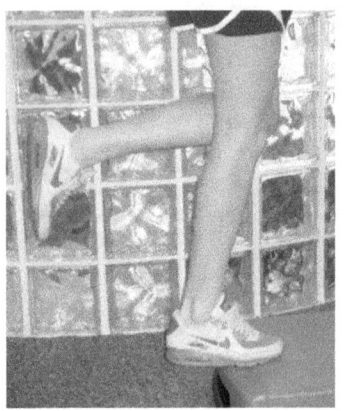 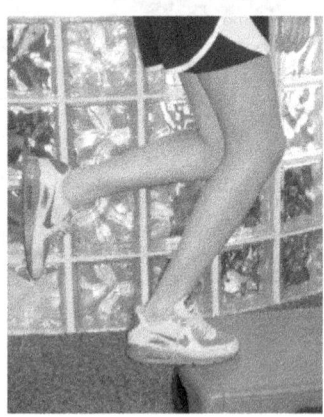

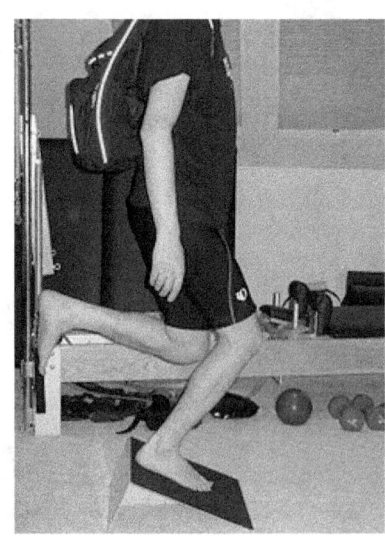

4. Towel Exercise: Before getting out of bed, with no shoes. Place a towel or resistance band around the bottom of your feet at the ball area. Pull on both ends of the towel/ resistance band while flexing your foot. Push your foot up and back 10 times, turn your foot to the right, flex your foot up and back 10 times in this position. Repeat for the other foot.

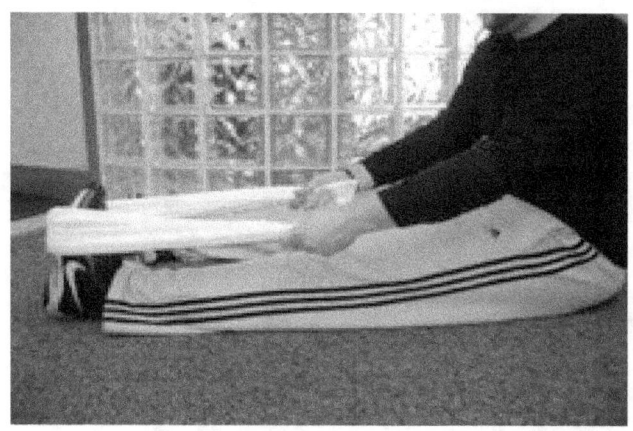

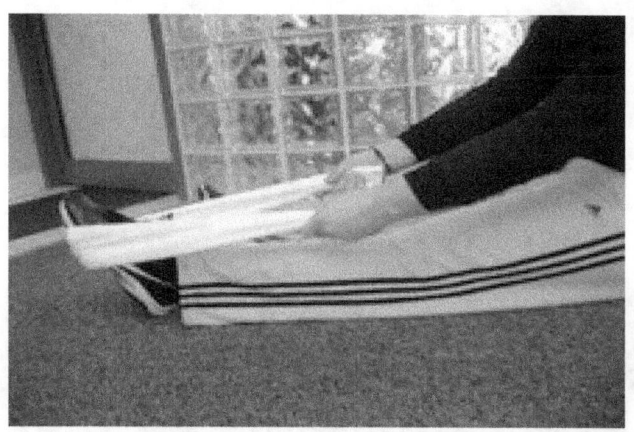

5. Step Drop: Begin by standing on a step or a stool with your heel hanging off. If you are using a stool, ensure that it is stable enough to hold your weight. You may need someone to hold the stool to stabilize it. Let your heels drop off the step 20 times. Repeat this exercise twice a day.

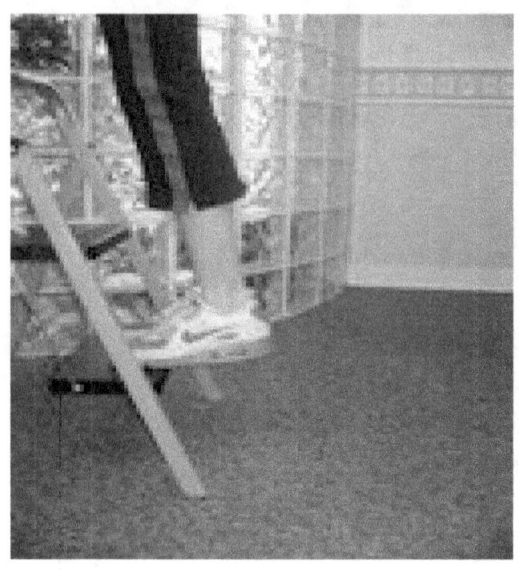

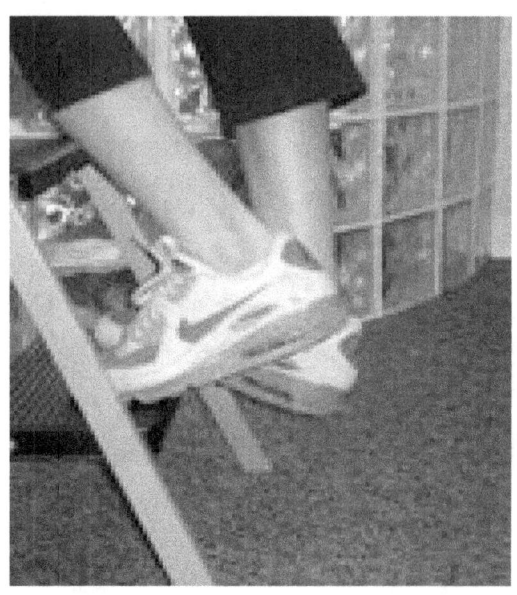

6. Toe Raises: Standing up straight, lift your heels so that your body is raised onto your toes. You may use a table or back of a chair for support. Start by doing 20 a day then add a few more each day. You will need to work up to doing 100 toe raises, twice a day.

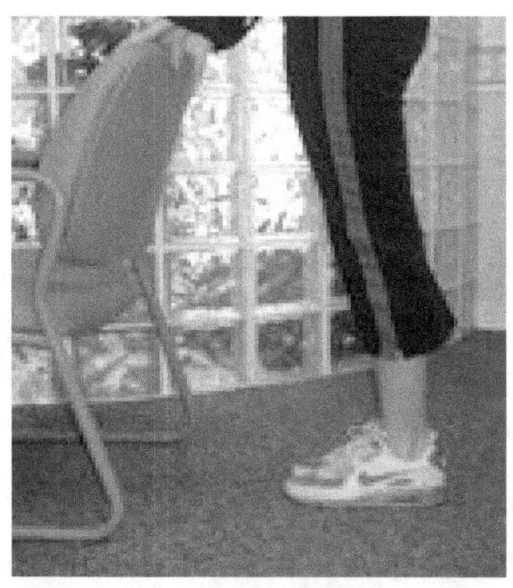

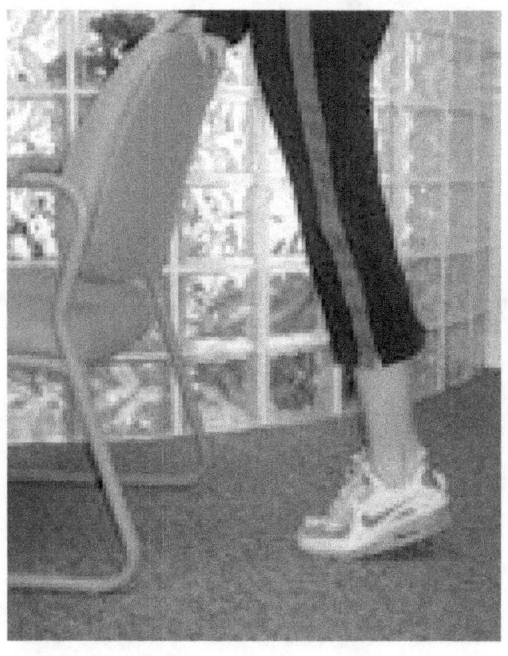

7. Foot Roll: A good exercise to reduce inflammation and relieve pain is to roll your foot on the Thera-Band Foot Roller (best and available in our office) or a frozen water bottle (wear socks and remember to only use a bottle ¾ full of liquid). This exercise should be done nightly. Repeat several times until you have relief.

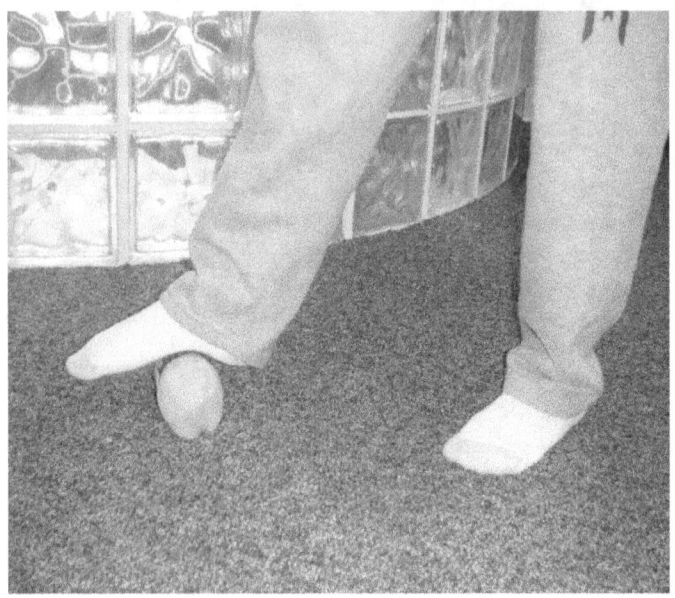

Conclusion

I hope you have enjoyed reading all of the articles in this book. Keep an eye out for my upcoming Weekend Doctor articles. Remember, if you are experiencing any foot pain do not hesitate to call your podiatrist. Foot pain is not normal and shouldn't have to get in the way of enjoying your life.

Sincerely,
Dr. Thomas F. Vail, DPM

www.ingramcontent.com/pod-product-compliance
Lightning Source LLC
Chambersburg PA
CBHW080259180526
45167CB00006B/2584